Adequacy of the VA Persian Gulf Registry and Uniform Case Assessment Protocol

Committee on the Evaluation of the Department of Veterans Affairs Uniform Case Assessment Protocol

Division of Health Promotion and Disease Prevention

INSTITUTE OF MEDICINE

NATIONAL ACADEMY PRESS
Washington, D.C. 1998

NATIONAL ACADEMY PRESS • 2101 Constitution Avenue, N.W. • Washington, DC 20418

NOTICE: The project that is the subject of this report was approved by the Governing Board of the National Research Council, whose members are drawn from the councils of the National Academy of Sciences, the National Academy of Engineering, and the Institute of Medicine. The members of the committee responsible for the report were chosen for their special competences and with regard for appropriate balance.

The Institute of Medicine was chartered in 1970 by the National Academy of Sciences to enlist distinguished members of appropriate professions in the examination of policy matters pertaining to the health of the public. In this, the Institute acts under both the Academy's 1863 congressional charter responsibility to be an adviser to the federal government and its own initiative in identifying issues of medical care, research, and education. Dr. Kenneth I. Shine is the president of the Institute of Medicine.

This study was supported by the Department of Veterans Affairs under Contract Number V101(93)P-1580. The views presented are those of the Institute of Medicine Committee on the Evalution of the Department of Veterans Affairs Uniform Case Assessment Protocol and are not necessarily those of the funding organization.

International Standard Book No. 0-309-06046-X

Additional copies of this report are available for sale from:

National Academy Press
2101 Constitution Avenue, N.W.
Box 285
Washington, DC 20055

Call (800) 624-6242 or (202) 334-3313 (in the Washington metropolitan area), or visit the NAP's on-line bookstore at **http://www.nap.edu.**

For more information about the Institute of Medicine, visit the IOM home page at **http://www2.nas.edu/iom.**

Printed in the United States.

The serpent has been a symbol of long life, healing, and knowledge among almost all cultures and religions since the beginning of recorded history. The serpent adopted as a logotype by the Institute of Medicine is a relief carving from ancient Greece, now held by the Staatliche Museen in Berlin.

COMMITTEE ON THE EVALUATION OF THE DEPARTMENT OF VETERANS AFFAIRS UNIFORM CASE ASSESSMENT PROTOCOL

Arthur K. Asbury, M.D. *(Chair),* Van Meter Professor of Neurology, Hospital of the University of Pennsylvania, Philadelphia

Dan G. Blazer, II, M.D., Ph.D., M.P.H., Dean of Medical Education and J.P. Gibbons Professor of Psychiatry and Community and Family Medicine, Office of the Dean, Duke University Medical Center, Durham, North Carolina

Dedra Stefanie Buchwald, M.D., Associate Professor, Department of Medicine, University of Washington, Harborview Medical Center, Seattle, Washington

Jerrold J. Ellner, M.D., Executive Vice Chair, Department of Medicine, Case Western Reserve University, Cleveland, Ohio

William E. Golden, M.D., Director, Division of General Internal Medicine, University of Arkansas for Medical Sciences, Little Rock, Arkansas

Bonnie Lepper Green, Ph.D., Professor of Psychiatry, Department of Psychiatry, Georgetown University Medical School, Washington, D.C.

Isabel V. Hoverman, M.D., Austin Internal Medicine Associates, L.L.P., Austin, Texas and Clinical Assistant Professor of Medicine, University of Texas Medical Branch, Galveston, Texas

Karl T. Kelsey, M.D., M.O.H., Associate Professor of Occupational Medicine, Harvard School of Public Health, Boston, Massachusetts

David L. Olive, M.D., Department of Obstetrics and Gynecology, Yale University School of Medicine, New Haven, Connecticut

Bernard M. Rosof, M.D., F.A.C.P., Senior Vice President, Medical Affairs, Huntington Hospital, Huntington, New York

Board on Health Promotion and Disease Prevention Liaison

Elena O. Nightingale,* Scholar-in-Residence, Institute of Medicine and Board on Children, Youth and Families, Washington, D.C.

Board on Neuroscience and Behavioral Health Liaison

William E. Bunney, Jr.,* Distinguished Professor and Della Martin Chair of Psychiatry, University of California, Irvine, California

Staff

Lyla M. Hernandez, Study Director
Donna D. Thompson, Division Assistant
Sanjay S. Baliga, Research Associate
Donna M. Livingston, Project Assistant
Kathleen R. Stratton, Director, Division of Health Promotion and Disease Prevention
Constance M. Pechura, Director, Division of Neuroscience and Behavioral Health

---

*Member Institute of Medicine.

Preface

This report is the third in a series of efforts by the Institute of Medicine to review the protocols used by the Department of Veterans Affairs (VA) and the Department of Defense (DoD) to diagnose the health complaints of Persian Gulf veterans. The first IOM review began in September 1994 and focused on the DoD implementation of the protocol which is referred to as the Comprehensive Clinical Evaluation Program (CCEP). This diagnostic protocol had been jointly developed and simultaneously implemented in mid-1994 by the VA and the DoD. The early initiation of this review provided the opportunity to analyze information on health complaints and programs collected from the very beginning of the implementation process. In January 1996, the committee issued a final report assessing the adequacy of the clinical procedures described in the protocol, and providing detailed recommendations to DoD for refining the original clinical approach.

The second IOM review initiated in July 1996 again focused on the DoD protocol, this time regarding the diagnosis of difficult-to-diagnose and ill-defined conditions, stress and psychiatric disorders, and health complaints that might be related to low-level exposure to nerve agents. Detailed information available from the existing data system was essential for conducting this evaluation on specific diagnoses in these areas. The final report was published in January 1998.

This third review differs from previous efforts in two key respects. First, this committee was charged with a much broader task. In conducting this review of the diagnosis of health problems of Persian Gulf veterans, we were asked to examine the VA health care delivery system, a system which differs markedly from that of DoD in both size and patient population. This analysis of the system included evaluating (1) the adequacy of the protocol as a diagnostic tool ***for the broad range*** of medical assessment needs of Persian Gulf veterans, not for specific clinical diagnoses, (2) how well the program was implemented including the process for patients referrals, (3) VA outreach activities, and (4) VA provider education.

The timing of this review is a second critical difference. Because the committee began deliberations in February 1997, almost two and a half years after the initial review of the DoD protocol, we had the opportunity to draw upon and benefit from both the IOM evaluations and additional information not heretofore available. For example, information was available reflecting nearly three years of VA experience in implementing the protocol, we could solicit new information from VA facilities regarding the strengths and challenges of the protocol, and we could draw upon recent research literature on health problems of Persian Gulf veterans and on advances made in developing clinical practice guidelines and pathways aimed at improving efforts to diagnose health complaints. The committee was, therefore, in an excellent position to evaluate the adequacy of the ***system*** used by the VA to identify and diagnose the health complaints of Persian Gulf veterans.

Thus, the recommendations of this report are different from those of previous reports, not only because of the much broader scope of the committee's charge, but also because of recent advances in clinical practice guidelines and quality evaluation approaches, and because of new information available to the committee about the strengths and challenges of the ongoing system. The earlier IOM studies provided important recommendations for implementing and improving the DoD and VA protocol. But any serious evaluation of an ongoing diagnostic screening program will lead, ultimately, to new and improved generations of protocols and systems. The timing and resources available to this committee allowed us to develop recommendations toward that end.

Arthur K. Asbury, M.D.
Chair, Committee on the Evaluation of the Department of Veterans Affairs Uniform Case Assessment Protocol

Acknowledgments

The committee wishes to express its appreciation to the many individuals who contributed in various ways to the completion of this project. Those who made time in busy schedules to meet with us during our VA facility site visits include Mack Anderson, Kimberly Arlinghaus, Donald Barnes, William Binkley, Tom Bird, Carol Bodenheimer, Thomas Bowen, Andrea Cohen, Tesfai Gabre-Kidan, Arnold Gorin, Larry Hawkins, Steve Hunt, Raye Hurwitz, Susan Killin, Shirley Laday-Smith, Sum Lee, Linda Lewis, Jeff Lindeman, Leonard Marcella, Miles McFall, Patricia Ordorica, Jaime Ortiz-Toto, Warrenson Payne, Tammy Porter, Ron Ratliff, Alfredo Rohaidy, Arthur Rosenblatt, Richard Schrot, B.J. Searles, Phillip Shenefelt, Richard Silver, Charles Smith, Glenn Smith, Philip While, John Wicher, Ruel Wiley, and Timothy Williams.

We are also grateful to the following individuals with whom the committee met or from whom information was received: Mark A. Brown, Joseph S. Cassells, Timothy Finnegan, Patricia Jones, Stuart Fleishman, Frances M. Murphy, George Poindexter, Joan P. Porter, Matthew Puglisi, and Joseph Violante. The committee also wishes to extend its thanks to the VA health care facilities and the veterans service organizations who responded to our request for information. We hope we have included all those who contributed to this project. Any omission is inadvertent.

This report has been reviewed by individuals chosen for their diverse perspectives and technical expertise, in accordance with procedures approved by the NRC's Report Review Committee. The purpose of this independent review is to provide candid and critical comments that will assist the authors and the IOM in making the published report as sound as possible and to ensure that the report meets institutional standards for objectivity, evidence, and responsiveness to the study charge. The content of the review comments and draft manuscript remain confidential to protect the integrity of the deliberative process. We wish to thank the following individuals for their participation in the review of this report: Mark R. Cullen, M.D., Yale University School of Medicine; Bernard D. Goldstein, M.D., UMDNJ-Robert Wood Johnson Medical School; John E. Helzer, M.D., University of Vermont College of Medicine; Richard T. Johnson, M.D., Johns Hopkins University School of Medicine; Joseph P. Newhouse, Ph.D., Harvard University; Herbert S. Rigberg, M.D., Health Services Advisory Group, Inc.; and M. Donald Whorton, M.D., M.P.H., M. Donald Whorton, M.D., Inc.

While the individuals listed above have provided many constructive comments and suggestions, responsibility for the final content of this report rests solely with the authoring committee and the IOM.

Contents

Adequacy of the VA Persian Gulf Registry and Uniform Case Assessment Protocol

Executive Summary

On August 2, 1990, Iraq invaded the independent nation of Kuwait and the Persian Gulf War began. Within 5 days the United States began to deploy troops, the number of which would ultimately reach almost 700,000, in Operation Desert Shield. Intense air attacks against Iraqi forces began on January 16, 1991 (Operation Desert Storm), and a ground attack was launched on February 24, 1991. Within 4 days Iraqi resistance crumbled. Following the fighting the number of U.S. troops in the area began to decline, and by June 1991 fewer then 50,000 U.S. troops remained.

Most troops returned home and resumed their normal activities. However, a number of those who had been deployed to the Persian Gulf began to report health problems that they believed were connected to their deployment. These problems included the symptoms of fatigue, memory loss, severe headaches, muscle and joint pain, and rashes.

In 1992 the Department of Veterans Affairs (VA) developed a Persian Gulf Registry to assist in addressing questions about the health concerns of Persian Gulf veterans. Queries about exposures, particularly those associated with oil well fires, were included as part of the history taking. With continuing concern about the potential health consequences of service in the Persian Gulf, the Department of Defense (DoD) and VA met in 1994, revised the clinical program, and implemented this revised approach to diagnose veterans' health complaints, called the Comprehensive Clinical Evaluation Program (CCEP) by

DoD and the Persian Gulf Registry and Uniform Case Assessment Protocol (UCAP) by VA.

The Persian Gulf Registry is a basic initial examination aimed at diagnosing veterans' health problems. If a veteran's complaint cannot be diagnosed through the Registry examination, he or she is referred to UCAP for specialty consultation and testing.

The President's Advisory Committee, the General Accounting Office, and the Office of Technology Assessment have evaluated these programs and have made recommendations on the basis of their reviews. In addition, the Institute of Medicine (IOM) has conducted assessments of and made recommendations regarding CCEP.

In September 1996 VA asked IOM to evaluate the adequacy of the UCAP and its implementation with specific emphasis on (1) the protocol, (2) its implementation and administration, (3) outreach efforts to inform veterans of available services, and (4) education of providers. A committee of experts met; heard presentations from many groups and individuals including VA, the President's Advisory Committee, the General Accounting Office, the American Legion, and the Disabled American Veterans; conducted site visits of VA health care facilities; and solicited written testimony from VA health care facilities and veterans service organizations.

A great deal of time and a great deal of effort were expended by VA in developing and implementing a diagnostic program for Persian Gulf veterans that could be conducted in all VA facilities, from small rural primary care facilities to large urban tertiary complexes. This effort was begun immediately upon the cessation of hostilities and attempted to build on lessons learned from past program efforts, for example, those directed toward Vietnam veterans' health concerns. The initial program was implemented in 1992 and the revised program was implemented in 1994, veterans were examined, and information about their symptoms and conditions was collected.

The information that has emerged from the diagnostic program, from research studies, and from the veterans themselves has helped indicate where changes and improvements in the Registry and UCAP can be made. Change is part of a natural evolutionary process in developing good screening instruments for diagnosis. This is not to imply that the first efforts were inappropriate but, rather, that time leads to new knowledge, which leads to the ability to improve.

Such is the case with the VA Persian Gulf protocol. Over time, information has been obtained that can be used to help identify areas where change in the protocol and its implementation will be of benefit. This report is intended to assist VA in that effort to improve. As an operational system, the Persian Gulf Registry and UCAP have provided the opportunity for observation, evaluation, and feedback aimed at improvement. That is what the committee has done—observed, evaluated, and reported.

The committee's first recommendations address the process for diagnosing Persian Gulf veterans' health complaints. These are followed by recommendations regarding implementation and administration and the quality of services rendered. Next come recommendations related to outreach efforts and provider education. Broad recommendations appear in boldface type, with the subentries indicating recommendations following from these broader recommendations.

FINDINGS AND RECOMMENDATIONS

Diagnostic Process

The diagnostic and referral process specified in *VA Manual M-10* is laid out as a two-stage protocol. The protocol specifies that if, after an initial history and physical with minimal laboratory testing (Registry; Phase I), a diagnosis is not made, the veteran is referred to the UCAP for specialist consultation and additional testing (Phase II). The division of the diagnostic process into two phases is, however, an artificial designation that does not accurately reflect the way in which medicine is traditionally practiced.

The committee found that the diagnostic process followed in some facilities does not adhere to the written protocol, rather it is more clinically based. For example, it was found that Registry (Phase I) evaluations are supplemented in some facilities by selected consultations and tests from the UCAP (Phase II). Although this approach may be clinically more appropriate and should be encouraged, it is not the process specified by the current protocol. Such deviation introduces the problem of inconsistency in evaluations across facilities as well as variation in data recording and reporting. This failure, in turn, works against achieving one of the purposes for which the system was developed, that is, to identify previously unrecognized major diagnostic entities that could provide an explanation for the symptoms commonly reported in Persian Gulf veterans with unexplained illnesses (*VA Manual M-10*; see Chapter 3).

The committee believes that the goal of implementing a uniform approach to the diagnosis of Persian Gulf veterans' health problems is admirable and should be encouraged. To accomplish that goal, the committee makes several recommendations.

1. The committee recommends that the diagnostic pathway, illustrated in Figure 1, for the evaluation and referral of Persian Gulf veterans' health problems be adopted and followed by providers in each VA facility.

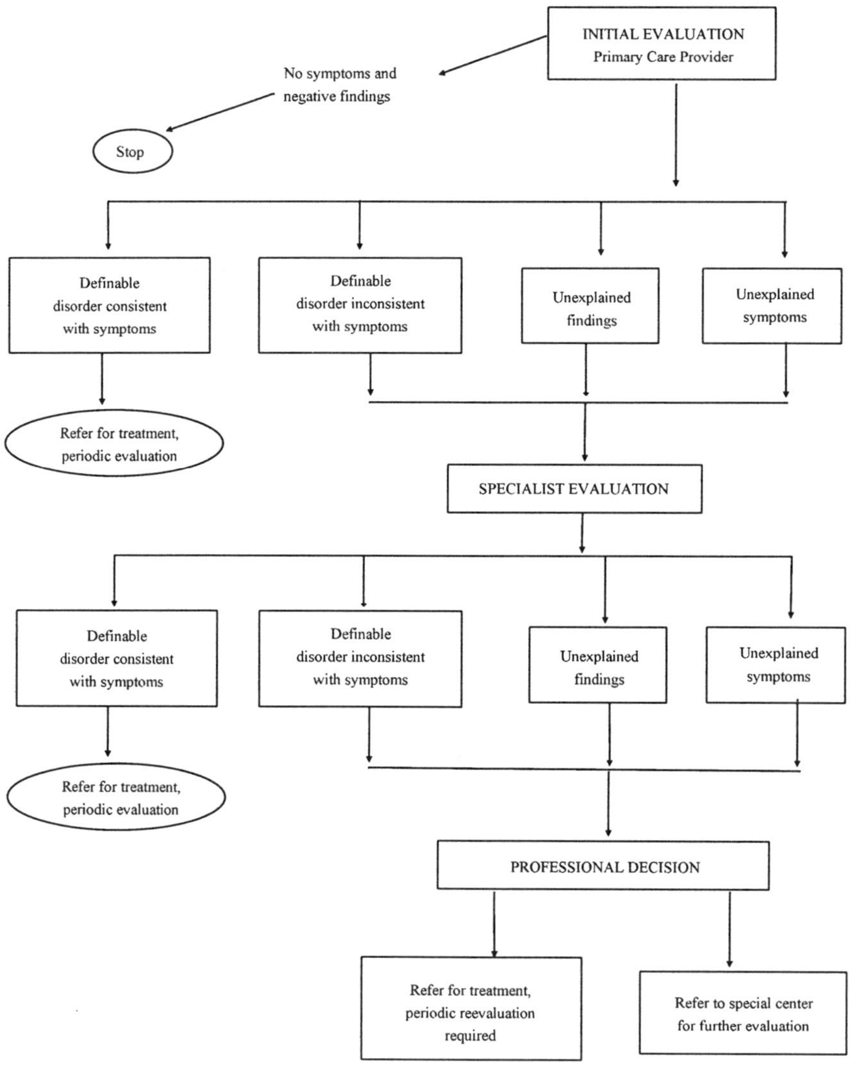

FIGURE 1. Pathway for diagnosing health problems of Persian Gulf veterans in the VA system.

The major differences between the current written protocol and the pathway recommended by the committee are (1) the primary care provider is encouraged to order additional tests and consultations beyond those specified in Phase I for a patient, based on symptoms and complaints, without the requirement of initiating a Phase II evaluation, (2) patients should be referred to a designated referral center only when the resources necessary to provide appropriate evaluation of presenting complaints are unavailable at the originating facility, and (3) there must be a defined approach to be used for patients who remain undiagnosed or whose major symptoms have not been accounted for (for example, periodic reevaluation, treatment, or referral to a referral center).

Adoption of the described pathway necessitates changes to specific elements of the Registry and UCAP protocols.

> 1.a. Use of the pathway eliminates the need to designate phases of evaluation; therefore, the distinction between Phase I and Phase II (with all accompanying specifications for specialty examination and referral) should be eliminated.
>
> > 1.a.(1) The Persian Gulf Registry Code Sheet needs to be redesigned to reflect the elimination of Phase I and Phase II from the protocol.
> >
> > 1.a.(2) The redesign should accommodate the need to aggregate data from the original data collection system with that of the redesigned system.

A minority of patients with persistent symptoms will not receive a definitive diagnosis. Some of these patients could have disease processes that cannot be diagnosed at present because of limitations in scientific understanding and diagnostic testing. They may not benefit from further evaluation now but may receive benefit from reassessment at a later date. This undiagnosed patient cohort, some of whom are designated as having an "unexplained illness," will contain a diversity of individuals who will require monitoring and periodic reassessment.

> 1.b. VA should plan for and include periodic reevaluations of the clinical needs of these undiagnosed patients.

The pathway specifies an initial evaluation by a primary care provider for both the veteran presenting with complaints and those with no complaints. In traditional medical practice, the comprehensive clinical evaluation of a patient presenting to any physician includes a complete history, physical examination, and laboratory tests. This should be no different for Persian Gulf veterans. The committee believes, however, that VA should consider using an expanded set of tests for the initial laboratory evaluation.

2. The committee recommends that both patients presenting with and those presenting without complaints should receive an initial evaluation which includes (1) a comprehensive history and physical as defined in the American Medical Association publication *Physicians' Current Procedural Terminology* (1998), (2) a very specific set of questions related to the Gulf War setting, and (3) a standardized laboratory evaluation.

> 2.a. A national panel of experts should be convened to (1) review the current set of Gulf War-related questions contained on the Persian Gulf Registry Code Sheet to determine whether additions or deletions are needed, (2) identify the set of standardized laboratory tests to be used in the initial evaluation, and (3) conduct periodic reevaluations of the usefulness of each element in the initial evaluation.

Specific Gulf War-related questions to which veterans are asked to respond include the exposure questions contained on the Persian Gulf Registry Code Sheet (see Appendix H). Given the importance placed by veterans and clinicians on the potential contribution of exposures to health complaints of Persian Gulf veterans, the committee decided to examine the exposure questions in detail.

At some facilities the questionnaire portion of this Code Sheet is given to the veteran to complete as a self-report form, whereas at other facilities this is completed during an interview with the provider. The committee believes that many of these questions are appropriate if administered by an interviewer but are not optimal as a self-report. The information collected with this questionnaire is not intended to be used for research purposes. Rather, the purpose of the questionnaire is to provide information to the clinician that might be used to assist in the diagnosis of health problems. It is important, therefore, that the patient understand what is being asked of him or her so as to provide the clinician with accurate information.

In addition, the questions related to traumatic experiences may miss important experiences that can affect physical and mental health and about which the physician should know when conducting the patient's evaluation.

> 2.b. The section on traumatic experiences on the Persian Gulf Registry Code Sheet (Question 19) should be expanded by the addition of (1) specific questions inquiring about experiences not presently assessed that have been reported by Persian Gulf veterans, and (2) an open-ended question(s) that allow(s) the veteran to report idiosyncratic or particularly distressing experiences that may play a role in the veteran's current health status.
>
> 2.c. The questionnaire should be administered in an interview format. If the information on environmental exposure, immunizations, and exposure

to traumatic situations cannot be collected in an interview format, all yes and don't know responses should be reviewed with the patient in a face-to-face evaluation.

When the Registry and UCAP protocols were developed, they were designed to be very broad and to capture as much information as possible about potential health concerns that could affect Persian Gulf veterans. The information collected through that system as well as the information obtained from other providers and through scientific studies allows efforts to be more appropriately focused on identifying and diagnosing Persian Gulf veterans' health problems. One mechanism that can aid these efforts is the development of clinical practice guidelines which are statements developed for the purpose of assisting the provider and the patient in making decisions about appropriate health care.

3. The committee recommends that VA, to the extent possible, use an evidence-based approach to develop and continuously reevaluate clinical practice guidelines for the most common presenting symptoms and the difficult-to-diagnose, ill-defined, or medically unexplained conditions of Persian Gulf veterans.

Because the Persian Gulf War was the first engagement in which women formed such a large proportion of deployed troops (7%) and because potential exposure of this group of women to stressors, reproductive system toxicants, and other health hazards may produce disorders distinct from those seen in prior conflicts, the committee believes that VA has a unique opportunity to examine the health of women deployed under such conditions. Therefore, there should be increased examination of and attention directed toward women's health issues. The current Registry and UCAP do investigate infertility or subfertility. However, evaluation of miscarriages, stillbirths, and congenital malformations and the evaluation of genitourinary or other hormonally related diseases are limited.

3.a. Clinical practice guidelines for the evaluation and management of women's health issues should be developed.

A major principle in the development and use of clinical practice guidelines is that there must be a mechanism that encourages feedback on the adequacy of the guidelines and their ease of implementation.

3.b. VA should develop a formal mechanism that enables practitioners to provide feedback on the practice guidelines and the diagnostic process used in the VA clinical program for Persian Gulf veterans.

Implementation and Administration

The committee focused its examination of the implementation and administration of the Registry and UCAP on four elements that it believes are of prime importance to the adequate functioning of the program. These four areas are (1) referral for specialty consultation both within and across facilities, (2) quality of services provided, (3) patient satisfaction, and (4) data collection and reporting.

Referrals

The committee found that problems often exist with referrals for specialty consultations. Within facilities, consultant practices are often booked weeks in advance resulting in long delays for specialty services. The referral specialist is frequently unaware that the referred patient is a Persian Gulf veteran, and the specialist may have little experience with the special needs and concerns of this group of patients. In addition, veterans undergoing this tertiary level of evaluation frequently have unrealistic expectations about the process and the outcome of their visit. One approach to addressing this problem is the use of clinical pathways which are clinical management tools that organize, sequence, and specify the timing of the major patient care activities and interventions of the entire interdisciplinary team for a particular diagnosis, procedure, or process.

4. The committee recommends that the process and procedures for referral be modified.

4.a. In those facilities where specialist consultations are provided, certain individuals within each specialty should be designated as the one(s) who will provide the consultative services to Persian Gulf veterans.
4.b. Clinical pathways should be developed to specify the events and processes involved in referrals for specialty consultation.
4.c. In the case of an inpatient evaluation, a site-specific clinical pathway should be used to facilitate the timely and efficient evaluation of patients.
4.d. The diagnostic pathway should specify that a patient be referred to another facility for evaluation only when the resources necessary to provide appropriate evaluation of the patient's presenting complaints are unavailable at the originating facility.
4.e. VA should develop a transfer protocol that specifies procedures for initial contact and scheduling as well as the materials and processes necessary for a transfer, for example, a full copy of the veteran's record to date including all laboratory tests and consultations, the differential diagnosis, and a procedure for the transfer of records from the tertiary

institution to the originating provider upon completion of the diagnostic workup.

Quality

There is a great deal of interest in and concern about the quality of care that Persian Gulf veterans are receiving in VA facilities. Although the VA has developed procedures for what it terms the Quality Management/Assessment Monitor (see Appendix K), this information is not adequate to evaluate the quality of care provided to Persian Gulf veterans. The committee believes that, overall, the clinicians involved in the VA Persian Gulf Registry and UCAP examinations are practicing medicine according to acceptable standards but there does not appear to be, across facilities, a systematic approach to documenting the quality of care provided or to identifying areas where improvement is needed.

Traditional quality improvement programs examined the structure within which care is provided, the process for providing care, or the outcomes of care in an attempt to identify the outliers or "bad apples." More recent approaches focus on performance improvement and are aimed at involving practitioners in the use of nonpunitive efforts that result in more effective changes and improvements to the system than was the case with approaches aimed at identifying practitioners with deficiencies.

The development and use of clinical practice guidelines, as recommended earlier, can be an important tool in a program for continuous quality improvement. Additionally, the participation of a multidisciplinary group of providers in the development of such guidelines increases the likelihood that needed changes will be more readily accepted.

5. The committee recommends that VA should establish an evaluation feedback mechanism that includes the elements of a performance improvement system.

Patient Satisfaction

The VA has implemented a well-developed and structured approach for assessing general patient satisfaction with VA care. However, there is no system in place specifically addressing the substantial number of issues and concerns specific and relevant to Persian Gulf veterans, or the special Persian Gulf diagnostic program.

6. The committee recommends that VA design and implement a brief yet comprehensive questionnaire to survey patient satisfaction with the special program for Persian Gulf veterans.

Data Collection and Reporting

An adequate and accurate data collection and reporting system is crucial to the understanding of Persian Gulf veterans' health problems. Such a system is needed to understand the extent of services provided, to contribute to assessments of the quality of services, to examine overall patterns in health status, and to contribute ideas for potential research studies that could be conducted on the health problems of Persian Gulf veterans. These data are not appropriate, however, for the conduct of scientific research.

Data collection forms need to be standardized and easily computerized. Those completing the forms should be doing so in a consistent manner from facility to facility. The committee found variation across sites in the diagnostic categories that practitioners used to identify their patients' health problems; for example, some practitioners use Chronic Fatigue Syndrome as a diagnosis and some do not. Additionally, the methods used to determine primary versus secondary diagnoses also appear to vary. Such variation has implications for the consistency and accuracy of data collection and reporting.

7. The committee recommends that VA facilitate the consistency of data reporting in the following ways.

7.a. There should be agreement nationally, within VA, on the definition and use of specific diagnostic categories.
7.b. Clear decision rules for determining and recording the primary diagnosis should be developed.

The committee also found that there was no opportunity for updating the database information gathered for each patient, even though a patient's condition can change in ways that are important for the analysis of information collected.

8. The committee recommends that there be established a mechanism by which individual patient information can be updated and incorporated in the database in a systematic fashion.

Outreach

The committee commends VA for the extensive effort it has put forth to inform Persian Gulf veterans of the services available to them. In only two areas has the committee identified needs.

9. The committee recommends that VA develop informational pamphlets for veterans. These pamphlets could be placed in facility treatment areas and could address common concerns such as the purpose and process of the VA Persian Gulf program, health effects of low-level exposure to chemical warfare agents, research activities related to Persian Gulf veterans and their results to date, and so forth.

When first entering a VA health care facility to receive services, all veterans complete an intake form that requests information about their service in the military. This presents an opportunity for the identification of Persian Gulf veterans who may not yet have participated in the special VA program for Persian Gulf veterans but who may wish to do so.

10. The committee recommends that VA consider redesigning intake forms so that the veteran is asked to identify whether or not she or he was deployed to the Persian Gulf War (or any other specific engagement).

Provider Education

VA has designed a number of high-quality programs to educate its designated Persian Gulf providers. These programs would be more effective if they reached a broader audience.

11. The committee recommends that primary care providers, in addition to the Registry practitioners, as well as the specialists who see Persian Gulf veterans, be provided the opportunity and encouraged to participate in the educational programs.

11.a. The audience for whom existing educational activities are developed related to providing health care for Persian Gulf veterans should be expanded to include other providers involved in the evaluation process, for example, designated specialty consultants.
11.b. VA should consider the following options for educating its providers: periodic team conferences (perhaps quarterly) to be held with all designated providers (including specialists) to discuss activities and findings and to provide updates on Persian Gulf issues and concerns, and the development of site-specific clinical pathways by designated specialists and Registry providers.

Although reproductive issues have been addressed in VA educational efforts, other women's health issues have been less thoroughly explored.

11.c. Future educational efforts should place greater emphasis on women's health concerns.
11.d. VA should provide resources to establish a repository for accumulated knowledge of, expertise in, and experience with the health issues and problems of Persian Gulf veterans. Specialists who possess such expertise should be identified and available for consultation by telephone, e-mail or telemedicine connections with local providers in all VA facilities.

TABLE 1. Summary of Recommendations

Topic	Recommendation
Diagnostic Process	**1. A national diagnostic pathway for evaluation of Persian Gulf veterans' health problems should be adopted.** 1.a. The distinction between Phase I and Phase II should be eliminated. 1.a(1). The Persian Gulf Registry Code Sheet needs to be redesigned to reflect the elimination of Phase I and Phase II. 1.a.(2) Provision should be made for the aggregation of data from both the original and the revised systems. 1.b. There should be a plan for periodic reevaluation of patients without a diagnosis.
	2. All patients entering the special VA program for Persian Gulf veterans should receive an expanded initial evaluation. 2.a. A national panel of experts should be convened to determine the specific questions and tests to be included in this expanded evaluation. 2.b. The section on exposures should be expanded to include additional questions about traumatic experiences. 2.c. The questionnaire should be administered in an interview format, but at a minimum, all yes and don't know responses should be reviewed with the patient.
	3. Clinical practice guidelines should be developed for the most common presenting symptoms and the difficult-to-diagnose, ill-defined, or medically unexplained conditions.

Continued

TABLE 1 *Continued*

Topic	Recommendation
Diagnostic Process (*cont'd.*)	3.a. Clinical practice guidelines for the investigation of women's health issues should be developed. 3.b. A formal mechanism that enables practitioners to provide feedback on the practice guidelines and their implementation should be developed.
Referral	**4. The committee recommends that the process and procedures for referral be modified.** 4.a. Within facilities providing specialty consultation, certain individuals within each specialty should be designated to provide consultative services to Persian Gulf veterans. 4.b. Clinical pathways should be developed to specify the events and processes involved in referrals for specialty consultation. 4.c. If an inpatient evaluation is conducted, a site-specific clinical pathway should be used to facilitate timely and efficient evaluation. 4.d. Patients should be referred to another facility for evaluation only when the necessary resources are unavailable at the originating facility. 4.e. A transfer protocol should be developed to facilitate referral to another facility.
Quality	**5. VA should establish an evaluation feedback mechanism that includes the elements of a performance improvement system.**
Patient Satisfaction	**6. VA should design and implement a brief yet comprehensive questionnaire to survey patient satisfaction with the special program for Persian Gulf veterans.**
Data	**7. VA should facilitate the consistency of data reporting in the following ways:** a. There should be agreement nationally, within VA, on the definition and use of specific diagnostic categories. b. Decision rules for determining and recording the primary and the secondary diagnoses should be developed **8. A mechanism to allow updating of individual patient information should be developed.**

Continued

TABLE 1 *Continued*

Topic	Recommendation
Outreach	**9. VA should develop for veterans informational pamphlets that address their concerns.** **10. Intake forms should be redesigned to more easily identify the war or conflict in which veterans served.**
Education	**11. Primary care providers, in addition to the Registry practitioners, as well as the specialists who see Persian Gulf veterans, should be provided the opportunity and encouraged to participate in the educational programs.** 11.a. The audience for whom existing Persian Gulf educational activities are developed should be expanded to include other providers involved in the evaluation process. 11.b. VA should consider as educational activities team conferences that include specialists and should consider development of site-specific clinical pathways. 11.c. Future efforts should place greater emphasis on women's health concerns. 11.d. Resources should be provided to establish a repository for accumulated knowledge, expertise, and experience in Persian Gulf health issues and problems.

SUMMARY

Change is inevitable and as such, it is important to plan for that change on the basis of new information and techniques that have emerged from past experiences. The committee believes that the changes recommended in this report build on the strengths and lessons learned through research, the implementation of the Registry and UCAP, and advances made in the field of clinical practice evaluation. It is with the intent to assist VA with better serving Persian Gulf veterans as well as facilitating the practice of VA practitioners that these recommendations are offered.

The committee believes that the recommendations contained in this report will clarify areas of confusion and engage VA practitioners in efforts to design practice guidelines and pathways that will result in the rendering of better, more timely diagnostic services to Persian Gulf veterans. The committee urges VA to make the implementation of these recommendations a priority.

1

Introduction

On August 2, 1990, Iraq invaded the independent nation of Kuwait. In rapid response the United Nations passed Resolution 678, which directed that "all necessary means" be used to get Iraq out of Kuwait. Within 5 days the United States had begun to deploy troops to the Persian Gulf in Operation Desert Shield. Intense air attacks against the Iraqi forces began on January 16, 1991 (Operation Desert Storm). A ground attack was launched on February 24, and within 4 days Iraqi resistance crumbled. Almost 700,000 U.S. troops participated in the Persian Gulf War. Following the fighting the number of U.S. troops in the area began to decline rapidly. By June 1991 fewer than 50,000 U.S. troops remained.

The demographic characteristics of the Persian Gulf troops differed from those involved in previous military engagements. Overall, they were older, a large proportion (about 17%) were from National Guard and Reserve units, and almost 7% of the total forces were women.

U.S. casualties during the Persian Gulf War were low. There were 148 combat-related deaths, with an additional 145 deaths due to disease or accidents. Despite the low numbers of U.S. fatalities and injuries, deployed personnel were exposed to a number of stressors. The rapid mobilization for military service led to the sudden disruption of the lives of large numbers of people. The involvement of large numbers of reservists and National Guard personnel created particular concern because in addition to their rapid mobilization and deployment, they would be returning directly to civilian life at the conclusion of the war.

Stressors to which U.S. troops were exposed included oil smoke, diesel and jet fuel, solvents and other petrochemicals, CARC (chemical agent resistant coating) paint, depleted uranium, sand, endemic infections such as leishmaniasis, the extreme heat, and primitive living conditions. In addition, some soldiers were given anthrax and botulinum vaccines and some soldiers ingested Pyridostigmine Bromide pills to protect against chemical warfare agents.

Other stressors affecting the troops were the unfamiliar character of the region, the requirement that U.S. military personnel have virtually no interaction with the indigenous populations, the wait for the fighting to begin, the fear that chemical warfare agents would be used by the Iraqis, and the immense destruction visited on the whole nation of Iraq, including exposure to dead and mutilated Iraqis.

After the war most veterans returned home and resumed their normal activities. Within a relatively short time, however, some active-duty military personnel and veterans began to report various health problems that they believed were connected to their service in the Persian Gulf. Symptoms commonly described included fatigue, memory loss, severe headaches, muscle and joint pain, and rashes (Iowa Persian Gulf Study Group, 1997).

In 1992, the Department of Veterans Affairs (VA) developed and implemented the Persian Gulf Registry. Its original purposes were to ease returning veterans into the VA health care system, to create a registry containing medical and other data on Persian Gulf veterans that would assist in addressing questions about possible future effects of air pollutant exposure and other environmental agents, and to serve as the basis for future medical surveillance. Exposures, particularly those associated with the oil well fires, were included as part of the history taking. As time passed it became apparent that a number of exposure issues and a host of symptoms needed further investigation.

As concern escalated over the health problems of those deployed to the Persian Gulf, the Department of Defense (DoD) also decided to develop and implement a Persian Gulf clinical program. DoD and VA met, used experts to develop clinical protocols, and by 1994 both had implemented similar and parallel clinical evaluation programs. VA's in-depth clinical program is called the Uniform Case Assessment Protocol (UCAP) whereas DoD's is called the Comprehensive Clinical Evaluation Program (CCEP).

By early 1994 over 20,000 veterans had been examined as part of VA's Persian Gulf Registry program. There were concerns, however, about whether those veterans were being appropriately diagnosed and cared for under the VA program. In response to those concerns, in 1994 the Congress passed P.L. 103-446 which stated: "In each year after the implementation of the protocol, the Secretary shall enter into an agreement with the National Academy of Sciences under which agreement appropriate experts shall review the adequacy of the protocol and its implementation by the Department of Veterans Affairs."

In September 1996, VA charged the Institute of Medicine (IOM) with evaluating the adequacy of the UCAP and its implementation. The expert

Committee on the Evaluation of the VA Uniform Case Assessment Protocol was convened to review the VA Persian Gulf clinical protocol and data collection, the adequacy of its implementation of the programs, outreach efforts to veterans, and the education of providers.

2

The Institute of Medicine's Persian Gulf Activities

IOM has undertaken several activities focusing on the potential health implications of deployment in the Persian Gulf War and on DoD and VA responses to health concerns. The IOM Medical Follow-up Agency examined the health consequences of service in the Persian Gulf and developed recommendations for research and information systems. The first report of that group (IOM, 1995) recommended that "The VA Persian Gulf Health Registry should be limited and specific to gathering information to determine the types of conditions reported. . . . There should be efforts to implement quality control and standardization of data collected by the registry." The report went on to recommend that improved publicity regarding the availability of the Registry was needed. For a complete list of recommendations, see Appendix A.

The second and final report of the Medical Follow-up Agency (IOM, 1996a) provides 16 recommendations, with accompanying findings, concerning research and information systems needed regarding the health consequences of service during the Persian Gulf War (see Appendix B).

In 1994, DoD asked IOM to assemble a group of medical and public health experts to evaluate the adequacy of the CCEP. That committee concluded that specific changes in the protocol would help increase its diagnostic yield but that, overall, the CCEP was a comprehensive effort to address the clinical needs of those who served in the Persian Gulf War. That report also stated that the CCEP was not appropriate as a research tool but that the results could and should be used to educate Persian Gulf veterans and the physicians caring for them, to improve the medical protocol itself, and to evaluate patient outcomes. (See Appendix C for a complete set of recommendations.)

DoD asked IOM to continue its evaluation of the CCEP giving special attention to three issues: (1) approaches to addressing difficult-to-diagnose individuals and those with ill-defined conditions, (2) the diagnosis and treatment of stress and psychiatric conditions, and (3) the assessment of health problems of those who may have been exposed to low levels of nerve agents. A report addressing the adequacy of the CCEP relative to nerve agents was released in April 1997 (IOM, 1997). It concluded that, overall, the CCEP provides an appropriate screening approach to the diagnosis of neurological diseases and conditions but that certain refinements would enhance the program. (See Appendix D for a complete set of recommendations.)

The issues of medically unexplained conditions and stress and psychiatric disorders were addressed in a separate and final report. That report concluded that information provided over time has led to the ability to focus CCEP evaluation efforts on emerging areas of importance. To that end the committee made several suggestions including the need to emphasize treatment of symptoms, whether or not a diagnosis has been determined; the need to provide increased screening for depression, traumatic exposure, and substance abuse; the importance of conducting an evaluation across facilities to determine consistency in terms of examinations and patterns of referral; and the need for greater communication between DoD and VA, particularly as it relates to the ongoing treatment of patients. A complete set of recommendations appears in Appendix E.

In September 1996, VA asked IOM to convene a panel of experts to fulfill the congressional mandate to review the VA Persian Gulf protocol and its implementation. Specific areas to be addressed included the adequacy of (1) the protocol to address the wide range of medical assessment needs of Persian Gulf veterans, (2) the implementation of the protocol and administration of the program, (3) outreach efforts to inform veterans of available services, and (4) education of providers.

Over the course of the project the committee heard presentations and reviewed written material provided by representatives of VA, the Presidential Advisory Committee, the General Accounting Office, the American Legion, and Disabled American Veterans. In addition, the committee reviewed the VA manual and protocol for the Persian Gulf Registry and UCAP; received reports of the health and research activities being undertaken in Britain and Canada regarding their Persian Gulf War veterans; examined the relevant scientific literature; solicited written input from national veterans organizations and all VA health facilities; conducted site visits to three VA facilities; and received staff updates on testimony, research, quality assurance activities, and other information related to the health of Persian Gulf veterans. This report contains the findings and recommendations of that committee.

3

The Department of Veterans Affairs Persian Gulf Registry and Uniform Case Assessment Protocol

This section of the report describes the special VA program designed to diagnose the health complaints of Persian Gulf veterans. The topics covered include the initial examination (the Persian Gulf Registry), the secondary level of examination (the UCAP), the process for referral, the data collection and reporting system, the designated VA providers and their responsibilities, the performance monitoring system, some descriptive statistics of program participants, VA outreach efforts, and VA provider education activities.

PERSIAN GULF REGISTRY

In 1992, VA implemented a program aimed at diagnosing the health problems of Persian Gulf veterans. In 1994, a revised VA clinical program for diagnosing the health problems of Persian Gulf veterans was implemented. This revised program is formally divided into two phases, the Registry examination (Phase I) and the UCAP (Phase II). During the Phase I Registry examination, (see Appendix F) a complete medical history is to be taken and is to include a family history; an occupational history; a social history including tobacco, alcohol, and drug use; a civilian history of possible exposures to toxic agents; a psychosocial history; and finally, a review of systems. The examiner is to record the time of onset of symptoms or condition, their intensity, the degree of physical incapacitation, and details of any treatment received. In addition, each veteran is to be given a complete blood count (CBC), an electrolyte glucose

(SMA-6, SMA-12) or equivalent blood chemistries and enzyme studies, and a urinalysis.

PHASE II: UNIFORM CASE ASSESSMENT PROTOCOL

The manual specifies that, "Individuals who after completing Phase I or Registry evaluations, have a disability and do not have a clearly defined diagnosis which explains their symptoms, must receive the following supplemental baseline laboratory tests and consultations." This level of examination is called Phase II or UCAP.

According to *VA Manual M-10*, "The concept behind the protocol was to identify previously unrecognized major diagnostic entities which could provide an explanation for the symptoms commonly reported in Persian Gulf veterans with unexplained illnesses." The protocol states that those referred to UCAP "must receive" the tests listed for the Phase II protocol. For example, all patients are to receive a set of supplemental baseline laboratory tests that include a CBC, Sedimentation Rate Erythrocyte Sedimentation Rate, C-Reactive Protein, Rheumatoid Factor, Anti-Nuclear Antibody, Liver Function, Creatine Phosphokinase, Hepatitis Serology, Human Immunodeficiency, VDRL, B-12 and Folate, Thyroid Function Test, Urinalysis, and Tuberculosis skin test Purified Protein Derivative.

In addition, the patient is to receive certain consultations including (1) dental, but only if the participant's annual screening is not done; (2) infectious disease; (3) psychiatry, but only with physician-administered instruments; and (4) neuropsychological testing, but only as indicated by a psychiatry consult. Additional examinations ordered are symptom-specific, that is, tests are specified based on the symptom(s). For example, if a patient complains of a headache, he or she undergoes magnetic resonance imaging and receives a lumbar puncture, which includes glucose, protein, cell count, VDRL, oligoclonal (IgC), myelin basic protein, opening pressure, and neurology. Other tests are required if patients exhibit other symptoms. (See Appendix G for the complete Phase II protocol.)

REFERRAL

If, after completing the UCAP investigation of the veteran's symptoms and conditions, a diagnosis is still elusive, the veteran may be referred to one of four Persian Gulf Referral Centers. The centers located in Washington, D.C., Houston, and Los Angeles were established in 1992, and the one in Birmingham, Alabama was established in 1995. The referral centers offer inpatient stays during which the veteran is observed, multidisciplinary consultations and serial physical examinations are conducted, and lengthy occupational and exposure histories are documented. Each center has available providers with clinical and academic expertise in multispecialty areas including pulmonary and infectious diseases, neurology, immunology, neuropsychology, and toxicology. Once veterans have completed their stay at the referral center, information is to be sent to the veteran's home VA medical center which is then to assume responsibility for providing follow-up care.

DATA COLLECTION AND REPORTING

A Persian Gulf Registry Code Sheet (see Appendix H) has been developed to collect basic information on all veterans seen through the Persian Gulf Registry, UCAP, or Referral Center evaluations. Part I of the code sheet is completed with the cooperation of the veteran and requests basic demographic information, exposure history, the veteran's evaluation of his own health status, and reproductive information. Part II of the Code Sheet is completed by the examining physician and requests information on symptoms, consultations needed, diagnoses, and the disposition of the patient (e.g., examination completed, hospitalized for future tests, or referred for outpatient care).

If UCAP is undertaken because of significant symptoms but no identifiable diagnosis, the remaining three pages of the Code Sheet are completed. The information requested on these pages includes tests performed, consultations completed, diagnoses made, and whether the physician believes that the veteran has an unexplained illness. A copy of each coded form is submitted to the Austin Automation Center, and the information on the form is entered into the computerized database. The original code sheet is to be filed in the patient's medical record. Copies are not returned to the medical center of origin unless corrections are required. The code sheets are then forwarded to the central VA headquarters in Washington, D.C. The information gathered by this process is to be analyzed for detection of patterns of disease.

In addition to the Persian Gulf Registry Code Sheet, a bimonthly report is required from all VA facilities (see Appendix I). This report provides statistical information on the total number of initial and follow-up examinations as well as cumulative totals, pending appointments, next appointment date, and number of missed appointments.

PERSONNEL

Each VA health facility is to designate a Veterans' Registry Physician (VRP) who is responsible for the clinical management of the Persian Gulf veteran and who serves as the primary health care provider until another one has been assigned. As defined in the VA manual, the major responsibilities of the VRP include (1) explaining the purpose of the physical examination to the veteran, (2) determining the focus of the initial examination and care provided for the symptomatic veterans, and (3) conducting and documenting the physical examination. This physician is also responsible for ensuring that a follow-up letter is mailed to each veteran explaining the results of the examination and laboratory tests (see Appendix J for sample follow-up letter).

In addition, each of the facilities is to have an identified Veterans' Registry Coordinator (VRC) who is responsible for the administrative management of the program including scheduling of appointments, monitoring time frame compliance, reviewing records for accuracy and completeness, and collecting data for the reporting process.

PERFORMANCE MONITORING

VA has developed an instrument (Appendix K) to be used "to assess and monitor the appropriateness of medical care being provided" through the Registry. Each VA medical center is to use the instrument to review at least 10% of its Registry examinations. The form elicits information on the required components of the Registry examination including the presence or absence of a Persian Gulf Registry Code Sheet in the health record; a "thorough history and physical exam such as completion of an SF88"; a breast examination and a gynecological examination for women; laboratory test results including CBC, blood chemistries, urinalysis, and chest X ray; record of follow-up visit; record of follow-up letter containing examination results and recommendations; and whether or not specific examinations were ordered if the veteran complained of persistent diarrhea, memory loss, shortness of breath, or chronic cough. A summary form for recording the monitoring results is also completed by each facility.

DESCRIPTIVE STATISTICS

Phase I Persian Gulf Registry examinations have been provided in 170 VA health facilities. Between August 1992 and May 1997, 67,989 veterans had received initial evaluations in these facilities. In September 1995 data began to be collected in such a manner that it became possible to identify whether veterans received Phase II examinations. From September 1995 to May 1997 data were collected on 5,970 patients. Of those patients, 695 received a Phase II examination and 422 patients were referred to one of the four Referral Centers for further evaluation.

Of the 5,970 veterans for whom data were collected on the revised Code Sheet, 90.2% were male and 9.8% were female. In addition, 70.6% were in active-duty units during the Persian Gulf War, 12.7% in Reserve units, and 11.1% were in the Guard; the unit status was unknown for 5.6% of those participating in the program. Most frequent complaints are listed in Table 3.1 while Table 3.2 lists the distribution of diagnoses.

TABLE 3.1 Most Frequent Complaints among 5,970 Patients

Complaint	Number	Percent
Loss of memory and other general symptoms	1,687	28.3
Headache	1,552	26.0
Fatigue	1,492	25.0
Muscle, joint pain	1,423	23.8
Skin rash	1,377	23.1
Sleep disturbances	718	12.0
Shortness of breath	679	11.4
Diarrhea and other gastrointestinal symptoms	657	11.0
Choking sensitivity	365	6.1
Chest pain	275	4.6
Abdominal	263	4.4
Other symptoms involving skin and integumentary tissue	244	4.2
Cough	222	3.7

TABLE 3.2 Distribution of Diagnoses among 5,970 Patients

Diagnosis	Number	Percent
Musculoskeletal and connective tissue	2,111	35.4
Mental disorders	1,909	32.0
Loss of memory and other general symptoms	1,687	28.3
No medical diagnosis	1,252	20.9
Skin and subcutaneous tissue	1,156	19.4
Respiratory system	1,120	18.8
Nervous system	1,022	17.1
Digestive system	971	16.3
Injury and poisoning	666	11.1
Circulatory system	613	10.3
Infectious diseases	538	9.0
Genitourinary system	333	5.6
Neoplasm	45	0.8

Information obtained from the VA on the 5,970 patients seen through May 1997 indicates that 80.1% of patients presenting with symptoms and examined through the Registry and UCAP received a diagnosis whereas 19.9% of patients with symptoms received no diagnosis. Of those who did not receive a diagnosis, 11.6% were classified as having an unexplained illness. An unexplained illness is defined by VA as "a single or multiple signs or symptoms which do not fulfill the definition of any conventional medical diagnosis but have a significant impact on the veteran's quality of life or functional status." It is possible, therefore, for an individual veteran to have symptoms but no diagnosis and not fulfill the criteria for unexplained illness.

OUTREACH

The Environmental Agents Service is the focal point within VA for clinical issues related to Persian Gulf veterans. It is from this office that many outreach efforts are organized and implemented. Extensive efforts have been expended to inform Persian Gulf veterans of the services available through the VA health care system. VA maintains a toll-free number (1-800-PGW-VETS or 1-800-749-8387) for persons with questions about Persian Gulf health issues, research findings, and applying for VA disability compensation. Veterans can request information over this automated helpline 24 hours a day, 7 days a week, or speak with a personal representative between 7:30 a.m. and 8:30 p.m. (central time). Helpline representatives encourage veterans to obtain a Registry examination. A VA Persian Gulf War veterans' illnesses home page is also available on the world wide web (http://www.va.gov/gulf.htm).

The primary vehicle for disseminating updated Persian Gulf War-related information to veterans is the *Persian Gulf Review* newsletter. This publication is produced three to four times annually and is sent directly to all Registry participants as well as to veterans who have asked to be placed on the mailing list. Approximately 180,000 veterans receive the publication, as do all VA medical centers, VA regional offices, and veterans' centers. To date, 14 issues have been published, the most recent being in September 1997. Other items produced for mass distribution include a brochure entitled "Persian Gulf Veterans' Illnesses: Questions and Answers" and a two-page fact sheet entitled "A Report to Veterans—Department of Veterans Affairs—Persian Gulf Research." A few facilities have developed their own brochures describing their programs for Persian Gulf veterans.

VA also offers an on-line bulletin board with updated information on Persian Gulf issues. On that bulletin board one may access the most recent issues of *Persian Gulf Review*, the most recent developments in Persian Gulf concerns, and facts about VA benefits and medical care for Persian Gulf War veterans.

PROVIDER EDUCATION

Extensive educational materials aimed at VA health care providers have been developed. The Environmental Agents Service periodically mails material related to Persian Gulf veterans' concerns directly to the Registry physicians and Registry coordinators in each VA health care facility.

Medical center staff also receive a substantial amount of information via interactive satellite teleconferences, interactive quarterly national telephone conference calls, and annual educational conferences. The most recent national conference on health consequences of service in the Persian Gulf War was held in early June 1997. This program covered a range of subjects related to Persian Gulf concerns (see Appendix L for a detailed agenda). In addition, a manual filled with reference material was distributed to each participant.

4

Committee on the Evaluation of the Department of Veterans Affairs Uniform Case Assessment Protocol

IOM was charged by VA with evaluating the adequacy of the UCAP, its implementation, VA efforts at outreach to veterans, and education of providers. IOM assembled a committee with expertise in neurology, neurobiology, internal medicine, infectious disease, gastroenterology, psychology, psychiatry, occupational and environmental medicine, obstetrics and gynecology, chronic fatigue syndrome, trauma, and clinical assessment. The full committee met three times, heard numerous presentations, and reviewed published material. In addition, the committee conducted site visits of VA health facilities to obtain firsthand information about the system and its implementation. The committee also solicited written testimony from VA health care providers and veterans service organizations on their views of the adequacy of the protocol and its implementation.

SITE VISITS

The committee determined that it was necessary to visit a range of VA health care facilities to understand how the providers at the local level are using the Registry and UCAP protocols, and implementing the program for Persian Gulf veterans. It must be emphasized that these visits were in no way intended to be a comprehensive survey of how the system was working. Rather, it was the intention of the committee to collect information that would provide a general picture of how individual VA health care facilities have organized to implement the protocols, and how the program was viewed by front-line providers in terms of its strengths and weaknesses.

The committee chose the sites to be visited primarily on the basis of geographic region and the total number of examinations of Persian Gulf veterans conducted. In addition, the committee decided that one of the facilities should be a referral center. With these general criteria in mind, the committee elected to visit (1) the VA Puget Sound Health Care System in Seattle, Washington; (2) the James A. Haley VA Medical Center in Tampa, Florida; and (3) the Houston Veterans Affairs Medical Center in Houston, Texas (a referral center).

Before the visits the committee developed a question guide for members to use during their visits. This guide was not meant to be an interview protocol but, rather, to serve as a reminder of the topics that committee members wished to cover during their visits to the facilities (see Appendix M for a list of the questions). Meetings were scheduled with (1) designated Persian Gulf Registry providers including physicians, nurse practitioners, and administrative staff; (2) specialists commonly called upon to see Persian Gulf veterans, for example, neurologists, psychiatrists, and dermatologists; (3) primary care providers (physicians, nurse practitioners, and nurses) who were *not* part of the Persian Gulf provider team but who would likely be involved in providing primary care to Persian Gulf veterans; (4) outreach personnel who were the first point of contact for the veterans and who conduct the local outreach activities; and (5) Persian Gulf veterans who were patients at the facility.

The committee divided into three subgroups to conduct the visits. Each subgroup consisted of at least two committee members plus one IOM staff person. All visits were conducted during April 1997 and each visit took two days. It was readily apparent that the Persian Gulf Registry and UCAP were implemented differently at each facility.

One facility had formed a Persian Gulf Clinic in which all Persian Gulf veterans receive the initial Registry and UCAP examinations as well as their follow-up care from a single physician. This physician integrates all of the medical and laboratory work conducted during both Phase I and Phase II examinations. Only when the provider/patient relationship is well established is primary care provided through a different clinic.

The second facility is organized so that Registry examinations are provided on certain days of the week by one of two designated physicians. The examinations are scheduled by a coordinator who arranges for the routine laboratory and X-ray studies to be carried out before the appointment. If the patient's first contact with the facility is through the Registry, the follow-up care is typically provided by one of the Registry physicians. It is not unusual, however, to assign patients to other primary care clinics for follow-up once the health Registry and UCAP examinations are completed.

In the third facility, all Phase I Registry examinations are conducted by a physician's assistant and are coordinated by the Registry physician. A social worker follows all Registry patients in an attempt to ensure that scheduled specialty consultations are completed and reported. Follow-up care is provided in the primary care clinics by other than the designated Persian Gulf providers. Referral center patients are generally cared for on an inpatient basis, with services coordinated by a designated physician. Follow-up care is provided at the home VA facility.

WRITTEN TESTIMONY

Letters were mailed to 167 VA health care facilities and to 37 veterans service organizations asking them to provide comments, based on their own experiences, about the adequacy of the VA Persian Gulf Registry and UCAP. Specifically, each was asked to submit written information that described its experience with the VA clinical program as it related to (1) the adequacy of the clinical protocol to address the wide range of medical assessment needs of Persian Gulf veterans, (2) how well the protocol had been implemented and administered by VA, and (3) the adequacy of education for providers and veterans about the program.

VA Health Facilities

Responses were received from 89 VA health care facilities. About one-third of those responding stated that the protocol was adequate, that it had been implemented and administered well, and that education for providers and veterans had been sufficient. The remainder of the responses provided more specific information on both the strengths and the challenges of the program. For a more complete summary of responses, see Appendix N.

High praise was given for the VA Environmental Agents Service educational efforts aimed at providers, including the annual national Persian Gulf Conference, video conferences, teleconferences, and newsletter updates, although many believed that the potential audience was much greater than the number of people who were currently participating.

Respondents reported difficulties regarding communication with and scheduling of specialty consultations and referral center visits, problems in completing the Registry Code Sheet, and reported the need for more information that could be distributed to the Persian Gulf veterans.

Overall, the respondents indicated they believed that the program was working fairly well in their own facilities, that minor adjustments were needed, and that they were committed to meeting the needs of their Persian Gulf veteran populations.

Veterans' Service Organizations

Five veterans' service organizations responded to the request for information. There were comments on a broad range of issues, some of which are beyond the scope of this IOM committee's charge, for example, funding levels for VA health care.

Regarding the Persian Gulf Registry and UCAP, VA was praised for its extensive efforts to inform Persian Gulf veterans of the existence of this program. Respondents also indicated that most Registry providers appear dedicated, concerned, and familiar with the program and Persian Gulf issues, in general.

Some expressed concern however, that although the VA protocol appeared appropriate for diagnosing common ailments, it did not appear effective for veterans with difficult-to-diagnose or ill-defined conditions. Although referral centers were established to aid in this area, only a small portion of those with undiagnosed illnesses are referred to such centers. Other respondents believed that there was a failure to pursue testing for possible causes of problems among the Persian Gulf veterans such as exposure to depleted uranium. It was suggested that chronic health problems may have led to poor mental health or depression that has gone unrecognized and not tested for in the VA protocol.

Respondents indicated that a major concern was that once patients receive a diagnosis and are referred for care, there is no assurance that follow-up care is received or is adequate.

5

Findings and Recommendations

DISCUSSION

VA has a large health care system, and as such, it not only reaps the benefits of but is also subject to the strains and limitations of any large organization. VA facilities run the gamut from the small rural primary care facility to the large urban tertiary care complex. It was for this system that an effort was undertaken to develop and implement a clinical diagnostic program that would identify the health problems of those who served in the Persian Gulf War and that could be implemented in each facility, regardless of its size. That effort was begun immediately upon the cessation of hostilities and drew upon lessons learned from past efforts to respond to the needs of Vietnam veterans.

A great deal of time and effort was expended to develop and implement a program that would provide high-quality diagnostic services to those deployed to the Persian Gulf. However, time brings new information and experiences that serve to indicate improvements that can be made. Change is part of a natural evolutionary process in developing good screening instruments and processes. This is not to imply that the first efforts were inappropriate but, rather, that time leads to new knowledge, which leads to the ability to improve.

Such is the case with the VA Persian Gulf protocol. Over time, information has been obtained which can be used to help identify areas where change in the protocol and its implementation will be of benefit. This report is intended to assist VA in that attempt.

The conclusions and recommendations reported here are not meant to serve as an indictment of the efforts of the VA providers who are working to provide high-quality services to the veteran population. Rather, as an operational system, the Persian Gulf Registry and UCAP provide the opportunity for observation, evaluation, and feedback aimed at improvement. That is what the committee has done—observed, evaluated, and reported.

The following section provides findings and recommendations, organized as follows. First, the committee provides its recommendation on the overall process to be used in a program focused on diagnosing Persian Gulf veterans' health problems. This is followed by specific recommendations regarding the elements of the process, its implementation and administration, and the quality of services rendered. Next come recommendations related to outreach efforts to veterans and provider education. Broad recommendations appear in boldface type, with subentries indicating recommendations following from these broader recommendations.

DIAGNOSTIC PROCESS

The diagnostic and referral process specified in *VA Manual M-10* is laid out as a two-stage protocol. The protocol specifies that if, after an initial history and physical with minimal laboratory testing (Registry; Phase I) the veteran does not receive a diagnosis, he or she is referred to UCAP (Phase II) for specialist consultation and testing. Division of the diagnostic process into two phases is, however, an artificial division which does not accurately reflect the way in which medicine is traditionally practiced.

The committee found that the diagnostic process followed in some facilities does not adhere to the written protocol but is, instead, more clinically driven. That is, evaluations as carried out in some facilities are often tailored to the symptoms and complaints of the patient, not blind adherence to the written protocol. Phase I evaluations in such facilities are frequently supplemented by selected consultations and tests from Phase II (e.g., the Registry provider does not wait until a Phase II designation to order pulmonary function tests if the patient complains of shortness of breath). It also appears that the entire Phase II protocol is not necessarily implemented in some facilities if a diagnosis that accounts for the primary complaints of the veteran can be arrived at without the full workup.

Although it is encouraging that providers are using their clinical judgment to evaluate veterans who present with symptoms, such practices result in confusion about where the patient is in the diagnostic process when compared to the written protocol mandated by VA. The current differentiation between a Phase I and a Phase II evaluation varies from facility to facility, that is, it depends on the facility in which a patient is examined rather than, as the protocol specifies, on whether the patient has received a diagnosis that explains his or her significant symptoms. Such variation introduces the problem of inconsistency in data recording and reporting across facilities, which, in turn, works against achieving one of the purposes for which the system was developed, that is, to identify previously unrecognized diagnostic entities that could provide an explanation for the symptoms commonly reported in Persian Gulf veterans with unexplained illness.

The committee believes that the desire to implement a uniform approach to the diagnosis of health problems in Persian Gulf veterans is admirable and should be encouraged. In order to accomplish this goal, however, the committee believes that several changes need to be made in the system. First, the system needs to be conceived of as a diagnostic pathway or process along which every patient flows. The committee believes that the following pathway (see Figure 5.1) provides the appropriate framework for clinical diagnosis and referral.

1. The committee recommends that the diagnostic pathway, illustrated in Figure 5.1, for the evaluation and referral of Persian Gulf veterans' health be adopted and followed by providers in each VA facility.

Following this pathway, a Persian Gulf veteran entering the system with no complaints would be given the initial evaluation as specified above, and if nothing was found upon examination and testing, that veteran's evaluation would stop. A veteran presenting with the complaint of diarrhea would be given the initial evaluation as specified above with the addition of such tests as stool examination and endoscopy. If the results of the examination and testing were consistent with a diagnosis that explained the complaints (for example, intestinal parasites), that patient's diagnostic evaluation would stop and she or he would be referred for treatment. If, however, the results were *not* consistent with the complaint or if something unexplained appeared as a result of the tests or the examination, the patient would continue on the diagnostic pathway for additional evaluation and testing. Eventually, if a diagnosis cannot be determined, the provider must decide whether (1) the symptoms or problems are serious enough to cause disruption in the patient's life and therefore warrant continued evaluation at a special center or (2) symptoms and complaints are not causing disruption in the patient's life and therefore the patient should receive periodic reevaluations to determine if his or her condition changes over time.

The major differences between the current written protocol and the pathway recommended by the committee are (1) the primary care provider is encouraged to order additional tests and consultations beyond those specified in Phase I for a patient, based on symptoms and complaints, without the requirement of initiating a Phase II evaluation, (2) patients should be referred to a designated referral center only when the resources necessary to provide appropriate evaluation of presenting complaints are unavailable at the originating facility, and (3) there must be a defined approach to be used for patients who remain undiagnosed or whose major symptoms have not been accounted for (for example, periodic reevaluation, treatment, or referral to a referral center).

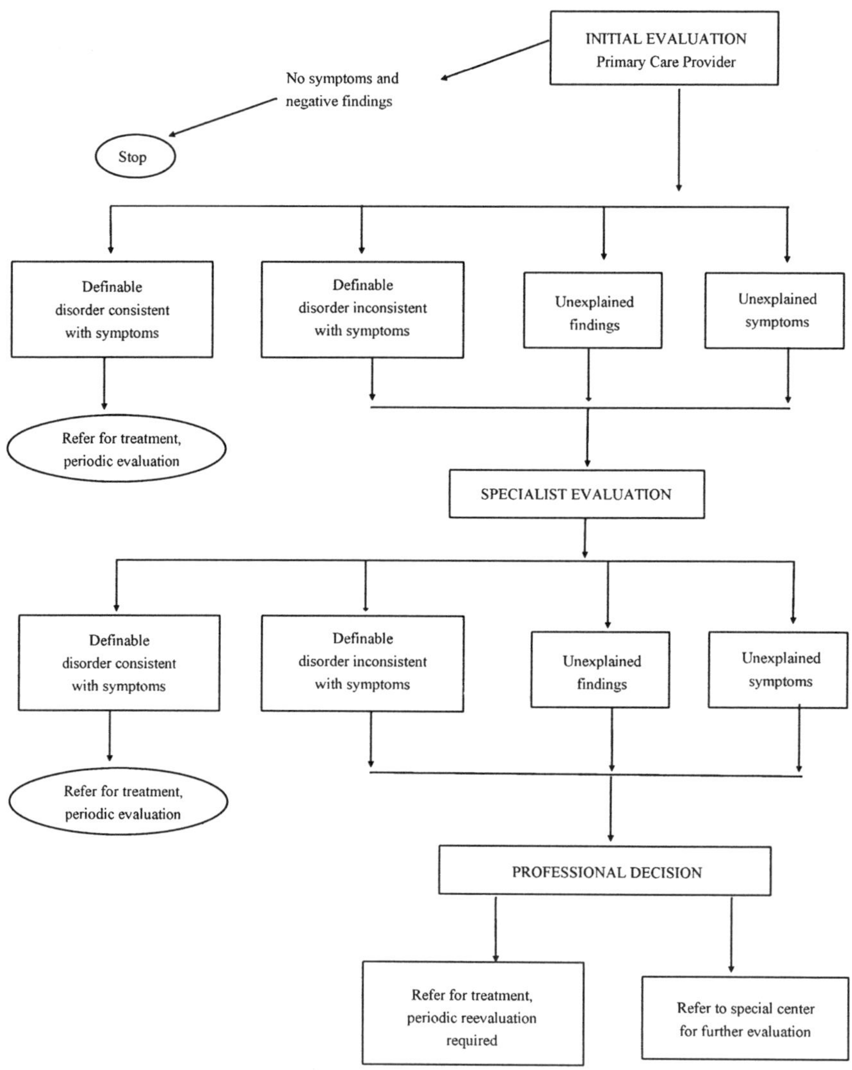

FIGURE 5.1. Pathway for diagnosing health problems of Persian Gulf veterans in the VA system.

Adoption of the described pathway necessitates specific changes to the protocols for conducting the Registry and UCAP examinations. A patient's position in the pathway is dependent upon whether the patient has received a diagnosis that accounts for his or her major symptoms. Although that was the apparent intent of the original protocols, the distinction between the Phase I Registry examination and the Phase II UCAP examination resulted in confusion among providers about which phase was being conducted and where information should be entered on the data recording form. If laboratory tests beyond those specified in the Phase I Registry (i.e., CBC, urinalysis, and blood chemistry tests) were ordered, did that mean that the patient was in Phase II? If a consultation with a neurologist was ordered, did that mean that the patient was in Phase II? Those questions are no longer relevant or important in the new diagnostic pathway.

1.a. Use of the pathway eliminates the need to designate phases of evaluation; therefore the distinction between Phase I and Phase II (with all accompanying specifications for specialty examination and referral) should be eliminated.

1.a.(1) The Persian Gulf Registry Code Sheet needs to be redesigned to reflect the elimination of Phase I and Phase II from the protocol.

1.a.(2) The redesign should accommodate the need to aggregate data from the original data collection system with that of the redesigned system.

A minority of patients with persistent symptoms will not receive a definitive diagnosis. Some of these patients could have disease processes that cannot be diagnosed presently because of limitations in scientific understanding and diagnostic testing. They may not benefit from further evaluation now but may receive benefit from reassessment at a later date. This undiagnosed patient cohort, some of whom are designated as having an "unexplained illness," will contain a diversity of individuals who will require monitoring and periodic reassessment.

1.b. VA should plan for and include periodic reevaluations of these undiagnosed patients' clinical needs.

The pathway specifies an initial evaluation by a primary care provider for the Persian Gulf veteran. In traditional medical practice, the comprehensive clinical evaluation of a patient presenting to any physician includes a complete history, physical examination and laboratory tests appropriate to the presenting complaints or clinical problems. This should be no different for Persian Gulf veterans. In addition, some veterans may not be experiencing difficulties but may wish to participate in the program. An initial evaluation with a basic set of elements should be given to both groups of patients, with additional tests performed as necessary based upon presenting complaints for those veterans with clinical problems or complaints.

The results of that initial evaluation will determine whether the patient proceeds further in the diagnostic process, as reflected in the recommended clinical pathway. The committee believes that VA should consider using an expanded set of tests and additional exposure questions for the initial evaluation.

2. The committee recommends that both patients presenting with and those presenting without complaints should receive an initial evaluation which includes (1) a comprehensive history and physical as defined in the American Medical Association publication *Physicians' Current Procedural Terminology* (1998), (2) a very specific set of questions related to the Gulf War setting, and (3) a standardized laboratory evaluation.

> 2.a. A national panel of experts should be convened to (1) review the current set of Gulf War-related questions contained on the Persian Gulf Registry Code Sheet to determine whether additions or deletions are needed, (2) identify the set of standardized laboratory tests to be used in the initial evaluation, and (3) conduct periodic reevaluations of the usefulness of each element in the initial evaluation.

Specific Gulf War-related questions to which veterans are asked to respond include the exposure questions contained on the Persian Gulf Registry Code Sheet (see Appendix H). Given the importance placed by veterans and clinicians on the potential contribution of exposures to health complaints of Persian Gulf veterans, the committee decided to examine the exposure questions in detail.

In some facilities the questionnaire portion of this Code Sheet is given to the veteran to complete as a self-report form, whereas in other facilities this is completed during an interview with the provider. The information collected with this questionnaire is not intended to be used for research purposes. Rather the purpose of the questionnaire is to provide information to the clinician that might be used to assist in the diagnosis of health problems. It is important, therefore, that the patient understand what is being asked of him or her so as to provide the clinician with accurate information.

With regard to Question 18 and its subsections, covering smoking and war-related toxic exposures, the committee believes that these questions are appropriate if administered by an interviewer, but not optimal as a self-report. Since this section is frequently handed to the veteran to be filled out as a self-report form, the extent to which responses are checked by an interviewer is not clear.

The instructions to skip over certain questions on items 18A to 18F (the smoking questions) are also confusing. The problems with questions 18G to 18Z have to do primarily with comprehension. Some of the options are not explained, so the veteran may respond negatively even if he or she has been exposed. For example, CARC is spelled out, but no description is provided. Likewise, exposure to depleted uranium and mustard gas may not be acknowledged if the veteran does not know how to tell if he or she might have been exposed. Although "don't know" is a valid option, the committee assumes that the examining physicians would want to know as much as possible about probable exposure. For this reason, the veteran should be able to discuss these possible exposures.

The primary problem with the questions related to traumatic experiences (items 19A to 19F) is that the questionnaire may miss important experiences or stressors that can affect physical and mental health, and about which the physician should know when doing the patient workup. Research has shown that stressors have been associated with major depression, substance abuse, and a variety of physical health problems, including immune system dysfunction.

With men and women serving together in a difficult situation such as war, a unique series of concerns emerges regarding the incidence of physical or sexual harassment or assault or both. Chapter 1 of *VA Manual M-10*, Part III identifies some special health needs of women veterans of the Persian Gulf including the long-term consequences of rape, other sexual assault, sexual harassment, exposure to combat during military service, or mistreatment as a prisoner of war. However, there is no specific reference to rape or abuse in the protocol history, and there is no routine evaluation of these activities in the absence of "reproductive health problems."

Veterans have indicated that seeing others dead (including Iraqi soldiers) is a very stressful experience. There may have been other frightening experiences that were relatively uncommon but that would be very upsetting and stressful if one were exposed to them.

There needs to be a way for veterans to report traumatic or stressful experiences to the clinician so that these experiences can be taken into account in evaluating a veteran's health complaints. Even less classically traumatic experiences such as harassment may play a role in health outcomes. An open-ended question(s) would also be useful for nonnormative, yet highly stressful, experiences. VA has a number of research centers with trauma specialists who could assist with the specific wording of such questions. Examples of such questions are given in Appendix O, some of which are taken from Southwick et al. (1997).

> 2.b. The section on traumatic experiences on the Persian Gulf Registry Code Sheet (Question 19) should be expanded by the addition of (1) specific questions inquiring about experiences not presently assessed that

have been reported by Persian Gulf veterans, and (2) an open-ended question(s) that allows the veteran to report idiosyncratic or particularly distressing experiences that may play a role in the veteran's current health status.

2.c. The questionnaire should be administered in an interview format. If the information on environmental exposure, immunizations, and exposure to traumatic situations cannot be collected in an interview format, all yes and don't know responses should be reviewed with the patient in a face-to-face evaluation.

In addition to discussion of the exposure questions, the committee focused on examining the list of the consultations and tests required by the UCAP protocol if a veteran presented with specific symptoms. At the time of its development the VA protocol was an appropriate attempt to collect a wide variety of information that covered all known potential health concerns that could affect Persian Gulf veterans. Much has been learned since it was first implemented. It is now known that certain symptoms (e.g., fatigue, memory loss, severe headaches, muscle and joint pain, and rashes) are commonly reported by these veterans. Now that this additional information is available, areas upon which to focus efforts at identifying and diagnosing health problems can be discerned. One mechanism that can aid in these efforts is the development of clinical practice guidelines.

Great strides in methods for developing clinical practice guidelines have been made in the past few years. Clinical practice guidelines are defined as systematically developed statements that assist the practitioner and the patient in making decisions about appropriate health care for specific clinical circumstances (Field and Lohr, 1990). Once developed, clinical practice guidelines can be used to assist clinical decision making by patients and practitioners, to educate individuals or groups, to assess and assure the quality of care, and to guide the allocation of resources for health care (Field and Lohr, 1992).

There are two major approaches to the development of practice guidelines. The first approach, the evidence-based approach, emphasizes the significance of the science base for guidelines and the use of quantitative modeling for estimating and comparing outcomes. The other approach emphasizes professional judgment in areas in which the science is weak or nonexistent (Field and Lohr, 1992). It may be that for some of the conditions being seen in the VA Persian Gulf program, a melding of experience and judgment with scientific evidence, where it exists, is the best possible approach.

Efforts are already under way for the development of practice guidelines in the VA health care system. In January 1997, VA distributed to all of its facilities clinical guidelines for major depressive disorder, posttraumatic stress disorder, and addictive disorder (Veterans Health Administration, 1997). These guidelines were developed by and for VA clinicians.

3. The committee recommends that VA, to the extent possible, use an evidence-based approach to develop and continuously reevaluate clinical practice guidelines for the most common presenting symptoms and the difficult-to-diagnose, ill-defined, or medically unexplained conditions of Persian Gulf veterans.

These guidelines need to be specific, comprehensive, and flexible enough to be useful in everyday clinical practice. Multidisciplinary groups of those providing care should be involved in the development process.

The Persian Gulf War differed from previous U.S. military engagements in that 7% of those deployed (about 49,000) were women. Potential exposure by this group of women to stressors, reproductive system toxicants, and other health hazards may produce disorders distinct from those seen in prior conflicts or among the men who served in the Gulf. The committee believes that VA has a unique opportunity to examine the health of women deployed under such circumstances. Therefore, there should be increased examination of and attention directed toward women's health issues. The current Registry and UCAP do evaluate infertility or subfertility among males and females, miscarriages, stillbirths, and congenital malformations.

The evaluation of genitourinary or other hormonally related disease is limited, however. Evaluation of this area in the current system is symptom-driven, allowing for errors of omission to be made in the absence of patient awareness. In addition, as discussed above, the special health needs of Persian Gulf veterans related to physical or sexual harassment and assault should be systematically addressed.

3.a. Clinical practice guidelines for the evaluation and management of women's health issues should be developed.

During the site visits and in the VA responses to requests for input, it was noted that no mechanism for providing feedback on the adequacy of the protocol and its use is available. For example, the current protocol states that every patient who is not diagnosed after Phase I and who presents with headache is to undergo magnetic resonance imaging of the head and receive a lumbar puncture. However, lumbar punctures are rarely ordered. Feedback from providers on the usefulness of the tests recommended for the diagnostic process and on the clinical practice guidelines once they are developed would provide important information on what changes, if any, should be made in the evaluation process.

3.b. VA should develop a formal mechanism that enables practitioners to provide feedback on the practice guidelines and the diagnostic process used in the VA clinical program for Persian Gulf veterans.

IMPLEMENTATION AND ADMINISTRATION

The committee focused its examination of the implementation and administration of the Registry and UCAP on four elements that it believes are of prime importance to the adequate functioning of the program. These four areas are (1) referral for specialty consultation, both within and across facilities, (2) quality of services provided, (3) patient satisfaction, and (4) data collection and reporting. The following sections discuss the committee's findings and recommendations for these four areas.

Referrals

According to information received by the committee, referrals for specialty consultation or to a Referral Center present problems. Within facilities, consultant practices are often booked weeks in advance, resulting in long delays for specialty services. Workup and consultant appointments are often at the convenience of the clinic or specialty service, without consultation with the patient about his or her availability. Appointments may be spread over days or weeks, requiring patients to return frequently to the VA facility. For all veterans this can be a lengthy and time-consuming process. For the employed veteran, this can create additional difficulties related to missed work, missed pay, and poor employee evaluation.

In addition, once specialty appointments are scheduled and the veterans are seen, the referral specialist is frequently unaware that the patient is a Persian Gulf veteran or the specialist has little or no experience with the particular needs and concerns of this group of patients. This may create the perception that the care being provided is less than adequate, whether or not such is the case.

It is also the case that veterans undergoing evaluations at a tertiary level often have unrealistic expectations of the process and the outcome of the visit. They are unaware that many of the same questions and tests that they have already undergone will be repeated and that the process is extremely time-consuming. This often results in frustration and anger, exacerbating an already sensitive situation.

One approach to addressing this problem is the use of clinical pathways which are clinical management tools that specify the various activities involved in a project from start to finish and the amount of time anticipated to complete each of the activities (Hoffman, 1993).

Clinical pathways organize, sequence, and delineate the timing of the major patient care activities and interventions of the entire interdisciplinary team for a particular diagnosis, procedure, or process, defining key processes and events in the day-to-day management of care and identifying expected outcomes. They should be developed locally, because they are specific to the particular setting and the team who uses them (Veterans Health Administration, 1997).

4. The committee recommends that the process and procedures for referral be modified.

> 4.a. In those facilities where specialist consultations are provided, certain individuals within each specialty should be designated as the one(s) who will provide the consultative services to Persian Gulf veterans.

Designated specialists should receive initial orientation concerning Persian Gulf War-related medical issues in their area of expertise.

> 4.b. Clinical pathways should be developed to specify the events and processes involved in referrals for specialty consultation.

Facilitation of the workup for Persian Gulf veterans is an important consideration. The evaluation should be done in a manner that is as timely, efficient, and convenient as possible. If travel, distance, time off from work, or other obstacles make completion of the evaluation as an outpatient too onerous for a given veteran, then preplanned, rapid inpatient evaluation may be considered.

> 4.c. In the case of an inpatient evaluation, a site-specific clinical pathway should be used to facilitate the timely and efficient evaluation of patients.

Referral to another facility presents additional problems, for both the veteran and the practitioners. For the veteran, referral to another center for specialty services often creates problems related to travel, time off from work, and family considerations. For the providers, there is frequently difficulty related to initial contact with the referral facility, unreturned calls, and an inability to obtain copies of reports. There may also be a lack of communication between the originating facility and the referral facility regarding proposed treatment and follow-up. In addition, there appears to be a great deal of inconsistency from facility to facility in terms of when it is deemed appropriate to refer a veteran for this tertiary level of evaluation.

> 4.d. The diagnostic pathway should specify that a patient be referred to another facility for evaluation only when the resources necessary to

provide appropriate evaluation of the patient's presenting complaints are unavailable at the originating facility.

4.e. VA should develop a transfer protocol that specifies procedures for initial contact and scheduling as well as the materials and processes necessary for a transfer, for example, a full copy of the veteran's record to date including all laboratory tests and consultations, the differential diagnosis, and a procedure for the transfer of records from the tertiary institution to the originating provider upon completion of the diagnostic workup.

Quality

There is a great deal of interest in learning more about the quality of care that Persian Gulf veterans are receiving in VA facilities. Although the committee believes that, overall, the clinicians involved in the VA Persian Gulf Registry and UCAP examinations are practicing medicine according to acceptable standards, there does not appear to be across facilities a systematic approach to documenting the quality of care provided to Persian Gulf veterans or to identifying areas where improvement is needed.

VA has developed procedures for what it terms the Quality Management/Assessment Monitor (see Appendix K). According to the manual, this form (VA Form 10-9009C-1) is to be used by VA medical centers "to assess and monitor the appropriateness of medical care being provided" through the Persian Gulf program. The form is to be used to abstract information from the charts of at least a 10% sample of all Persian Gulf Registry physical examinations conducted at each facility. Unfortunately, the form only collects such information as whether an examination was done or ordered, whether laboratory results were obtained, and whether follow-up letters are in the record or were mailed to the veteran. This information does not represent an adequate assessment of the quality of care provided to Persian Gulf veterans.

In 1990, IOM defined quality of care as "the degree to which health services for individuals and populations increase the likelihood of desired health outcomes and are consistent with current professional knowledge." (Lohr, 1990).

Traditional quality assurance programs examined the structure within which care is provided, the process for providing care, or the outcomes of care in an attempt to identify the outliers or "bad apples." Current approaches focus on performance improvement and are based on a set of principles for implementing change. Their aim is to involve practitioners in the use of nonpunitive tactics for quality assurance that result in more effective changes and improvements to the system than was the case with traditional approaches that were aimed at identifying the practitioners with deficiencies.

The principles for performance improvement models emphasize the relationship between the partners in the health care transaction, the fact that errors are more often the result of defects in the system rather than individual deficiencies, the use of statistical and scientific precepts and techniques, reliance on self-improvement as opposed to external regulation, standardized processes, the provision of feedback to practitioners on their pattern of practice as compared to that of their peers, a visible commitment to quality by top leadership, and a striving for continuous improvement as opposed simply to the achievement of preset goals (Field and Lohr, 1992).

The development and use of clinical practice guidelines, as recommended earlier in this report, can be an important tool in a program for continuous quality improvement. Such guidelines can clearly define what is appropriate care, what are acceptable outcomes, and the contributions of practitioners and patients to those outcomes. These guidelines can be used to help structure the medical review criteria used to collect data on how the system is operating. Additionally, the participation of a multidisciplinary group of providers in the development of clinical practice guidelines increases the likelihood that needed changes will be more readily accepted.

5. The committee recommends that VA should establish an evaluation feedback mechanism that includes the elements of a performance improvement system.

Patient Satisfaction

The VA health care system, as is the case with any health care system that diagnoses and manages medical problems, must attend not only to objective outcomes (e.g., morbidity and mortality) but also to more subjective ones such as patient satisfaction. In fact, the measurement of patient satisfaction, as pioneered by the Medical Outcomes Study (Rubin et al., 1993), has become one of the most widely used and important outcomes both in the clinical arena (e.g., in assessing the success of interventions and other aspects of health care delivery) and in the health services research arena. The many questions that have arisen regarding the health consequences of the Persian Gulf War experience, coupled with widespread publicity on a myriad of potential adverse medical outcomes, make patient satisfaction a critical component of any evaluation of the adequacy of the UCAP.

VA has implemented a well-developed and structured approach for assessing general patient satisfaction with the care provided at VA facilities. However, no system specifically addressing the substantial numbers of issues and concerns specific and relevant to Persian Gulf veterans or the special Persian Gulf diagnostic program is in place.

6. The committee recommends that VA design and implement a brief yet comprehensive questionnaire to survey patient satisfaction with the special program for Persian Gulf veterans.

An example of the kind of instrument that might be developed can be found in Appendix P.

Data Collection and Reporting

An adequate and accurate data collection and reporting system is crucial to the understanding of Persian Gulf veterans' health problems. One explicitly stated purpose of the VA Persian Gulf Registry and UCAP is the creation of a registry that contains medical and other data on Persian Gulf veterans. This registry would assist in identifying previously unrecognized major diagnostic entities that could provide an explanation for the symptoms commonly reported in Persian Gulf veterans with unexplained illnesses (*VA Manual M-10*, Part III, Chapter 3, page 3-1). Toward that end, VA has established a database that is meant to be comparable and retrievable across VA health care facilities. These data are not, however, intended to be used for scientific research, nor are they adequate for the conduct of scientific research.

Because VA has only partially automated inpatient record-keeping, current on-line retrieval of data is not possible. However, VA has plans for construction of a computerized database for outpatient records. This should facilitate the review of any data collected through the Persian Gulf program.

Data collection and reporting should, in general, be completed by using standardized and field-tested instruments. The data should be recorded on forms that are easily computerized. Individuals completing the reporting forms should be trained in how to do so to ensure standardization of the quality of data collected across sites. Any data entry should be done in a systematic fashion, with routine error checking involved, and double entry should be used whenever possible. Error rates should be checked and reported. Frequent data quality meetings across VA sites would be advantageous for ensuring standardization.

Finally, the goals of all data collection and data reporting must be explicit and must be the guiding principle behind their development. That is, each data collection system and each system of reporting must be completed with specific goals in mind. This will provide a means for the evaluation of the success and of the strengths and weaknesses of this approach.

The Persian Gulf Registry and UCAP have been established by VA with the intent of implementing a uniform and consistent evaluation across facilities. Data are available; that is, medical records of Gulf War veterans are complete and have been recorded. However, with respect to the application of the medical protocols, standardization and reporting are problematic.

As discussed earlier, current evaluation of the patient tends, in many facilities, to proceed along medically indicated lines rather than being strictly protocol-driven. Thus, it is clear that there is little consistency with respect to designation of phase of evaluation. Such variation hampers evaluation efforts based on these reported data.

Until the national diagnostic pathway has been implemented, Phase I and Phase II eliminated, and the Code Sheet revised to reflect such changes, it is anticipated that this variation will continue.

The committee found that there was variation across sites in the diagnostic categories that practitioners used to categorize patients' health problems. Providers at some facilities used such diagnostic categories as chronic fatigue syndrome and fibromyalgia, while providers at other VA health facilities did not. Such variation in the use of diagnostic categories has implications for the consistency and accuracy of data collection and reporting.

Further, the method used to determine primary versus secondary diagnoses varies. While a primary diagnosis is to be recorded on the code sheet, no instructions are given regarding how to determine which diagnosis is primary. The committee found that some physicians list a medical diagnosis as primary over a psychiatric diagnosis. Other physicians do not follow this custom. Such variation introduces uncertainty about the consistency of the data.

7. The committee recommends that VA facilitate the consistency of data reporting in the following ways.

7.a. There should be agreement nationally, within VA, on the definition and use of specific diagnostic categories.
7.b. Clear decision rules for determining and recording the primary and the secondary diagnoses should be developed.

The committee also found that there was no opportunity for updating the database information gathered for each patient. That is, intake questionnaires and data gathered at the presentation of the patient cannot be updated later in any systematic fashion. This is true for both patients who receive a diagnosis and those who remain symptomatic but undiagnosed. A patient's health status can and does change over time, and the system must have some way of capturing that new information.

8. The committee recommends that there be established a mechanism by which individual patient information can be updated and incorporated in the database in a systematic fashion.

This includes revision of original diagnoses and revision of status including data that are related to life style or demographics.

OUTREACH

For Persian Gulf veterans to participate in the special program that VA has designed to address their health concerns, they must be aware that the program exists and know how to register for it. The committee commends VA for the extensive outreach efforts put forth to inform Persian Gulf veterans of the services available to them. As described earlier, the toll-free number (1-800-PGW-VETS or 1-800-749-8387) for those with questions about Persian Gulf health issues, the newsletters, the pamphlets, and the computer bulletin board (http://www.va.gov/gulf.htm) are designed to provide a number of venues through which veterans can obtain information.

However, there does appear to be a lack of reliable, easily understood information for Persian Gulf veterans regarding exposures and their health consequences. This information needs to be readily accessible and available.

9. The committee recommends that VA develop informational pamphlets for veterans. These pamphlets could be placed in facility treatment areas and could address common concerns such as the purpose and process of the VA Persian Gulf program, health effects of low-level exposure to chemical warfare agents, research activities related to Persian Gulf veterans and their results-to-date, and so forth.

When a veteran first visits a VA health care facility, she or he completes what is known as an intake form. Such forms in general use throughout the VA system are not designed to easily identify Persian Gulf veterans. Although intake forms request dates of active-duty service, no questions specifically ask whether the veteran served in the Persian Gulf War. Unless veterans so identify themselves, those performing the intake function would have to know about the VA Persian Gulf Registry *and* specifically ask about service in the Persian Gulf War. It is unlikely that this occurs, and therefore, an opportunity to identify veterans who may wish to participate in the program is lost.

10. The committee recommends that VA consider redesigning intake forms so that the veteran is asked to identify whether or not she or he was deployed to the Persian Gulf War (or any other specific engagement).

PROVIDER EDUCATION

One of the charges to the committee was to determine the adequacy of the provider education activities for those who participate in the diagnosis of Persian Gulf veterans' health problems.

As discussed earlier in the report, VA has designed a number of programs to educate its designated Persian Gulf providers including interactive satellite teleconferences, quarterly national telephone conference calls, direct educational mailings, and an annual conference on health consequences of service in the Persian Gulf War.

The committee was impressed with the high quality of these efforts, hopes that those for whom they have been designed avail themselves of the opportunity to participate, and believes that the audience who receives such education needs to be expanded.

Although the designated Persian Gulf providers are given the opportunity to participate, other primary care personnel and specialists do not usually receive the materials nor do they participate in the educational programs. Some specialists appeared to know little about the VA Persian Gulf Registry and UCAP, had little or no orientation to the program, and were unable to identify whether the patients whom they saw were Persian Gulf veterans. Although a number of educational opportunities to learn about the program exist (e.g., the yearly national conference, quarterly newsletters, conference calls, and videotapes), participation in such activities appears to be limited to the designated Registry providers.

11. The committee recommends that primary care providers, in addition to the Registry practitioners, as well as the specialists who see Persian Gulf veterans, be provided the opportunity and encouraged to participate in the educational programs.

> 11.a. The audience for whom existing educational training activities are developed related to providing health care for Persian Gulf veterans should be expanded to include other providers involved in the evaluation process, for example, designated specialty consultants.

The specialists with whom the committee spoke and those from whom the committee received input often felt frustrated that veterans sometimes appeared more knowledgeable about the latest Persian Gulf veterans' health issues and research results than they were. Many believed that such a lack of information could be interpreted as a lack of caring or a lack of expertise in treatment and could lead to patient dissatisfaction with the services he or she is receiving, even if those services were of high quality.

This lack of knowledge undermines Persian Gulf veterans' confidence in the system, worsening patient satisfaction and heightening public concerns about the adequacy of the VA system for addressing the health issues of Persian Gulf veterans.

The lack of in-depth involvement of the specialists also means that they do not have access to continuing medical education opportunities related to Persian

Gulf veterans' health issues and that they may not participate in an evaluation-feedback mechanism to determine the value of various parts of the protocol or system. The specialists are the ones ordering, providing, and evaluating the more sophisticated tests conducted during the evaluation process. They are in an excellent position to determine how appropriate or beneficial these might be for individual patients. Such feedback could be collated to look more closely at the tests that do result in some positive information about the nature of veterans' complaints.

> 11.b. VA should consider the following options for education of its providers: periodic team conferences (perhaps quarterly) to be held with all designated providers (including specialists) to discuss activities and findings and to provide updates on Persian Gulf issues and concerns; and development of site-specific clinical pathways by designated specialists and Registry providers.

Reproductive issues have been addressed in the educational efforts of VA. Although these concerns seem to have been discussed, aspects of health unique to women have been given a lower profile.

> 11.c. Future educational efforts should place greater emphasis on women's health concerns.

A tremendous amount of knowledge about the diagnosis and treatment of Persian Gulf veterans' health problems is being amassed in various sites around the country. It behooves VA to identify where and with whom this special expertise exists and to develop mechanisms whereby others can benefit from the lessons that have been learned.

> 11.d. VA should provide resources to establish a repository for the accumulated knowledge of, expertise in, and experience with the health issues and problems of Persian Gulf veterans. Specialists who possess such expertise should be identified and available for consultation by telephone, e-mail, or telemedicine connections with local providers in all VA facilities.

6

Conclusion

Change is inevitable, and as such, it is important to plan for that change on the basis of new information and techniques that have emerged from past experiences and scientific investigation. The committee believes that the changes recommended in this report build on the strengths and lessons learned through research, the implementation of the Registry and the UCAP, and advances made in the field of clinical practice evaluation. It is with the intent to assist VA with better serving Persian Gulf veterans that these recommendations are offered.

The committee believes that the recommendations to adopt the described diagnostic pathway, to eliminate the distinction between Phase I and Phase II, to add to the collection of exposure information, and to develop appropriate clinical practice guidelines and pathways with feedback mechanisms on their usefulness will facilitate better and more timely provision of diagnostic services to Persian Gulf veterans. The concomitant changes in data collection and reporting and the collection of information on patient satisfaction will elicit information that can be used to assist in focusing efforts aimed at continuously improving the system. It is important to note that the system remains a diagnostic program, not a research study, and it is therefore not reasonable to expect the Registry and UCAP to identify a new syndrome or syndromes. The current excellent approaches to outreach and provider education will be supplemented by the committees' recommendations for the exploration of additional avenues and the involvement of additional practitioners.

Although it will take thoughtful effort and time to plan for and implement these recommendations, the committee urges VA to make the implementation of these recommendations a priority.

References and Selected Bibliography

American Medical Association. 1998. Physicians' Current Procedural Terminology. Chicago: American Medical Association.

Field, M.J., and Lohr, K.N., eds. 1990. Clinical Practice Guidelines: Directions for a New Program. Washington, D.C.: National Academy Press.

Field, M.J., and Lohr, K.N., eds. 1992. Guidelines for Clinical Practice: From Development to Use. Washington, D.C.: National Academy Press. GAO (General Accounting Office). 1997. Gulf War Illness: Improved Monitoring of Clinical Progress and Reexamination of Research Emphasis Are Needed. Washington, D.C.: Government Printing Office.

Hoffman, P.A. 1993. Critical Path Method: An Important Tool for Coordinating Clinical Care. Joint Comm J Qual Improv 19:235–246.

Horne, M. 1996. Involving Physicians in Clinical Pathways: An Example for Perioperative Knee Arthroplasty. Joint Comm J Qual Improv 11:115–124.

IOM (Institute of Medicine). 1995. Health Consequences of Service During the Persian Gulf War: Initial Findings and Recommendations for Immediate Action. Washington, D.C.: National Academy Press.

IOM. 1996a. Health Consequences of Service During the Persian Gulf War: Recommendations for Research and Information Systems. Washington, D.C.: National Academy Press.

IOM. 1996b. Evaluation of the U.S. Department of Defense Persian Gulf Comprehensive Clinical Evaluation Program. Washington, D.C.: National Academy Press.

IOM. 1997a. Adequacy of the Comprehensive Clinical Evaluation Program: Nerve Agents. Washington, D.C.: National Academy Press.

IOM. 1997b. Adequacy of the Comprehensive Clinical Evaluation Program: A Focused Assessment. Washington, D.C.: National Academy Press.

Iowa Persian Gulf Study Group. 1997. Self-reported illness and health status among Gulf War veterans: A population-based study. JAMA 277(3):238–245.

Lohr, K.N., ed. 1990. Medicare: A Strategy for Quality Assurance, 2 vols. Washington, D.C.: National Academy Press.

Presidential Advisory Committee on Gulf War Veterans' Illnesses. 1996. Final Report. Washington, D.C.: U.S. Government Printing.

Rubin, H.R., Gandek, M.S., Rogers, W.H., Kosinski, M.A., McHorney, C.A., and Ware, J.E., Jr., 1993. Patients' Ratings of Outpatient Visits in Different Practice Settings: Results from the Medical Outcomes Study. JAMA 270(7):835–840.

Southwick, S.M., Morgan, C.A. 3rd, Nicolaou, A.L., and Charney, D.C. 1997. Consistency of memory for combat-related traumatic events in veterans of Operation Desert Storm. Am J. Psychiatry 154(2):173–177.

Veterans Health Administration. 1997. Clinical Guideline for Major Depressive Disorder (MDD), MDD with Post Traumatic Stress Disorder (PTSD), and MDD with Substance Abuse (SA). Washington, D.C.: Veterans Health Administration.

Appendix A

Health Consequences of Service During the Persian Gulf War: Initial Findings and Recommendations for Immediate Action*

FINDINGS AND RECOMMENDATIONS

In this report, the IOM Committee has attempted to highlight issues we believe would benefit from immediate action. In reviewing the large volume of documents and the progress of research currently underway, we have identified areas that need prompt attention. As the scope and extent of health problems of Persian Gulf veterans have appeared to expand, the social response also has grown. The committee believes that this has resulted in a fragmented attempt to solve these problems. Thus we believe that sustained, coordinated, and serious efforts must be made in the near term to focus both the medical, social, and research response of the Government and of individuals and researchers. Hence, the findings and recommendations that follow are offered with the intent to focus and sharpen the debate, and to improve the quality of the data, and thereby, scientific inference. Finally, we hope to impact in a positive way the health in persons who served in the Persian Gulf War, as well as in those who may follow in other military encounters.

Recommendations for immediate action follow based on the findings presented here and the background information presented in the next chapter. The recommendations are to be viewed as independent, and are not presented in

---

*This appendix was excerpted from the Institute of Medicine report *Health Consequences of Service During the Persian Gulf War: Initial Findings and Recommendations for Immediate Action,* Washington, D.C.: National Academy Press, 1995.

any priority order within categories. The recommendations are divided into three categories: data and databases, coordination/process, and considerations of study design needs.

DATA AND DATABASES

Finding I

The VA Persian Gulf Health Registry is not a population database and is not administered uniformly, therefore, it cannot serve the purposes of research into the etiology or treatment of possible health problems. The Committee recognizes that certain tabulated descriptions of affected persons may legitimately be carried out for reasons other than the generation of scientific data. Specifically, there may be medical reasons for collecting information about patients with certain kinds of problems, especially diagnostic problems, particularly in medical settings where the information may be subjected to more intense scrutiny. An example is the establishment of the VA referral centers for Gulf War veterans. Since a limited number of veterans have been referred to these centers, and because the sample is self-selected, the Committee concludes that it is unlikely that productive scientific research (especially of an epidemiological nature) can ever be based on the data generated by the referral centers or the health registry as currently organized.

Recommendations

- The VA Persian Gulf Health Registry should be limited and specific to gathering information to determine the types of conditions reported. The role of this registry should be clearly defined as a means for identifying and reporting illnesses among Gulf War veterans with concerns about their health. There should be efforts to implement quality control and standardization of data collected by the registry from other VA facilities. The VA registry data should not be promoted or described as a means to determine prevalence estimates or identify the etiology of a disease, but should be reviewed promptly for enrollment trends and potential sentinel events.
- The VA should improve publicity regarding the existence of the Persian Gulf Health Registry, and encourage all concerned PGW veterans to be registered.
- Where possible the referral centers, standardized protocol should be used in each VA facility.
- The timeliness of data received from the VA Medical Centers (VAMC) to be entered into the PG Health Registry database needs to be improved.

Finding 2

No single comprehensive data system exists that enables researchers to track the health of Persian Gulf War veterans both while on active duty and after separation. As a result, it is not possible to conduct research and determine the morbidity and mortality experience of this population. Although both the VA and the DoD have medical records systems in place, they are inadequate and unlinked. This lack of a single data system is a hindrance to research concerning delayed health effects, both for Persian Gulf veterans and for those serving in future encounters.

Recommendation

- The Vice President of the United States should chair a committee composed of representatives from HHS, DoD, and the VA to devise a plan to link data systems on health outcomes with the development of standardized health forms, the ability to access information rapidly, and an organized system of records for rapid entry into the data system.

Finding 3

The characteristics of the population at risk are critical to any definitive studies of Gulf War health effects. The DoD has taken the proper steps to enumerate and describe this population that will be part of the planned, but yet incomplete, Army Geographical Information System model.

Recommendations

- The DoD registry needs to be completed as quickly and accurately as possible.
- The secretaries of DoD and VA should develop a single service-connected health record for each present active duty and former service member. All health data entries should be recorded in this single record for the individual.

COORDINATION/PROCESS

Finding 4

The committee has noted with interest and some concern the wide variety of disciplines and expertise among persons who have considered possible causes of a mystery illness. It has appeared to the committee that some of these persons and organizations are simply not qualified to draw reasoned scientific conclusions, or to implement those conclusions by means of specific medical intervention. There may be substantial risk from inappropriate interventions because of adverse reactions to drugs, development of resistant strains of microorganisms, or especially the diversion of attention away from more orthodox diagnoses and treatments that hold some promise of relief from symptoms of a "mystery illness."

Recommendation

- Decisions to provide funding, to refer patients, or to change usual operating procedures for providing financial support should be based on more solid scientific bases than has sometimes been evident in prior resource allocation. Funding should be subject to external peer review and approval.

Finding 5

There are dozens of studies of PGW health effects under way now, and many others are being initiated. Several efforts appear to be redundant, yet there are clearly gaps where research efforts are necessary. In its final report, the IOM Committee will recommend some additional specific research projects.

Presently, the total number of undiagnosed conditions is unknown because the data either are insufficiently understood or unavailable. Data that are available are fragmented, managed by different methods in different agencies, and based on a wide variety of unconnected rationales, from both military and civilian institutions. Many research efforts should, but do not, rely on a common set of data resources. Because so many unanswered questions remain concerning multi-system etiologies that have been proposed to explain undiagnosed signs and symptoms, all future as well as current evaluations must ensure that findings can be reconciled across studies.

Recommendations

• The Persian Gulf Veterans Coordinating Board (chaired by the secretaries of VA, DoD, HHS) should actively coordinate all studies developed from any new initiatives that receive federal funding, to prevent unnecessary duplication and to assure that high priority recommended studies be conducted. These studies should undergo appropriate external peer review before, during, and after data collection and analysis.

• More staff should be assigned by the Persian Gulf Veterans Coordinating Board in order to monitor, collect, assemble, and make accessible when appropriate all relevant requested emerging data from studies now underway, and make periodic reports to the appropriate federal oversight authority.

• Each new initiative should be evaluated in the context of what it can contribute. That is, each new study should add something of value to the information already being obtained or accumulated.

CONSIDERATIONS OF STUDY DESIGN NEEDS

Finding 6

To date, most studies of PGW veterans have been piecemeal—one military unit here, one collection of volunteers with some problem there, etc. But, some of these studies have several fundamental problems. They are necessarily incomplete, they usually lack proper controls, they are hard to generalize, they are subject to grave statistical problems because of post-hoc hypotheses and multiple comparisons, and where an effect truly exists they tend to have low statistical power to detect a difference. Thus, bits and pieces are not likely to answer any critical questions. The committee recognizes that an initial effort to survey a sample of veterans is underway, but more is needed.

Overall, there has been a broad and serious lack of adequate attention to the design of individual studies, and even more seriously, the scope and organization of an appropriate collection of studies, each focused on the resolution of a specific question. The committee regards this as a grave, though understandable, failure. Experts in research design can and should work shoulder to shoulder with experts in the subject matter of each individual study; this is particularly true for work in epidemiology. A broader view of the whole collection of studies, including input from experts in subject matter and in research methods, persons knowledgeable about data sources and medical care systems, and those with general appreciation of public concerns and public policy, has been conspicuously lacking. We believe that good studies could be done, but that they will require substantial input from experts in epidemiological methods.

Recommendations

- The VA and DoD should determine the *specific* research questions that need to be answered. Epidemiologic studies should be designed with the objective of answering these questions given the input of experts in epidemiologic research methods and data analysis, along with the input of experts in the subject matter areas to be investigated.
- To obtain data on symptom prevalence, health status, and diagnosed disease, the secretaries of DoD and VA should collaborate to conduct a population-based survey of persons who served in the PG, and of PG-era service personnel. The study should be designed to allow for adequate comparisons of outcome by sex, service branch, and rank, with oversampling among certain subgroups to allow for analysis. The IOM committee is willing to comment on and assist in the study design. An evaluation of the feasibility and need for a longitudinal study should take place coincident with this national survey.

Finding 7

Initial characterizations of smoke and unburned contaminants from the oil well fires and other sources are not adequate, nor have the data available been reduced to a format usable for drawing conclusions or conducting health studies. Considerable data exist from a wide number of sources, but they have not been compiled or analyzed in any organized or efficient way. For example, lead levels that would cause acute toxicity have been reported; however, questions about the validity of these reports have not been adequately addressed.

Recommendations

- DoD should assemble and organize these data from all sources for evaluation by the IOM committee.
- DoD should conduct a study that simulates exposure in tents heated by diesel fuel, with composition similar to that used in the PG. Fuels and conditions should simulate as closely as possible the conditions that existed in the PG. Exposure to lead and its possible effects should be explored further. The committee reviewed work done indicating that some personnel in the Gulf had lead levels consistent with acute intoxication. Thus in investigating lead exposure, special attention should be given to any history of abdominal pain or mental disorders.

Finding 8

As acknowledged by the investigator, the VA study of mortality in the PG veteran population is of insufficient duration to observe a higher rate of death than would be expected from chronic disease outcomes.

Recommendation

- The VA should plan and provide support for its mortality study to continue in the future in order to permit the detection and investigation of long-term mortality from chronic disease.

Finding 9

Although infertility, unrecognized and recognized pregnancy loss, premature delivery, fetal growth retardation, birth defects, and abnormal development are all components of reproductive health, studies and surveillance efforts to date have focused primarily on birth defects, fetal and neonatal deaths, and low birth weight. Adverse reproductive effects can be mediated through males as well as females, so it is important to study exposures of both parents. Information on infertility and miscarriage has not been included in the VA Health Registry efforts. Moreover, data on outcomes are available only from a single cluster study in Mississippi and the Army Surgeon General's preliminary data evaluation. DoD recently launched a study of reproductive health, and the VA and DoD clinical evaluation protocols provide some surveillance of infertility, miscarriage, birth defects, and infant deaths.

The design of scientific studies to address reproductive risk associated with environmental exposures is complex. A variety of endpoints may occur throughout the continuum beginning with fertility, through intrauterine, peripartum, and neonatal development, and continuing with effects manifested only later in childhood. Additionally, sophisticated expertise is required to document environmental exposures as the etiology for adverse pregnancy experience. There are research groups in some academic and federal settings that could, if deemed appropriate, conduct such complex research.

Recommendations

- VA and DoD should include reproductive outcomes among the array of health endpoints in surveillance programs based on medical records and individual questionnaires. Medical records, such as those to be included in the Seabees reproductive study and the DoD reproductive health study, would be suitable to ascertain stillbirth, low birth weight, preterm delivery, and major birth defects. Questionnaires such as those administered for the VA health registry exam could, in addition, address questions of infertility and clinically recognized miscarriage.

• The Persian Gulf Veterans Coordinating Board should consider specific exposures that are most likely to adversely affect reproductive health of women, men, or both, distinguishing between agents that would affect reproductive health only if exposure occurred at or around the time of critical periods during pregnancy versus those that might have effects that would persist after the cessation of exposure. As specific hypotheses linking exposure and reproductive outcomes are identified, studies that are suitable to providing more conclusive results for those associations should be designed.

• The Persian Gulf Veterans Coordinating Board should remain alert but skeptical about cluster studies such as those underway in Mississippi. Studies of this kind may be valuable in suggesting etiologic hypotheses; however, they have little promise for resolving questions about links between experiences in the Persian Gulf and reproductive health. Population-based studies of reproductive health outcomes are essential to resolve questions of effects of Persian Gulf War service.

Finding 10

Women who did not realize that they were pregnant at the time were deployed to the Gulf; others became pregnant during their service in the Gulf. These groups of women may have been exposed to substances potentially hazardous to themselves and to their unborn babies. A study would permit comparisons of birth outcomes and potential adverse health effects on women exposed at different times in their pregnancies.

Recommendation

• The Persian Gulf Veterans Coordinating Board should conduct a study to compare women deployed to the PG who were or who became pregnant at any time during the Persian Gulf War with an appropriate group of other women who were pregnant, but did not serve in the PGW, to evaluate potential adverse health outcomes to the mother or child. This study should only be done if a sufficient number of women can be identified. Efforts should be made to gather exposure information relevant to service at potentially high-risk times during gestation.

Finding 11

The committee has become aware that rosters exist that contain the names of persons vaccinated with anthrax and botulinum toxoid.

Recommendation

- DoD should maintain its lists of those receiving anthrax and botulinum vaccines for the purpose of conducting follow-up studies on these cohorts.

Finding 12

Troops were given packets of pyridostigmine bromide (PB) pills to be taken as a prophylactic to the threat of nerve agent exposure, at the direction of their commanding officer. PB by itself, in recommended doses, is a safe drug. Additionally, DEET (*N,N*-diethyl-*m*-toluamide) and permethrin were used by the troops to prevent insect bites. There is some information about the possible long-term toxicity to humans of DEET absorbed through the skin; however there appears to be little or no information about dermal absorption of permethrin from residues left on clothing, bedding, or elsewhere. Although permethrin is generally not applied to skin, animal studies have shown that permethrin is transferred from cloth to skin, and subsequently absorbed (NRC, 1994). There is little information about how PB, DEET, and permethrin might interact; interactions among these compounds are possible and are inadequately studied.

Recommendation

- Studies are needed to resolve uncertainties about whether PB, DEET, and permethrin have additive or synergistic effects. Unsubstantiated suggestions that they may have chronic neurotoxic effects need to be tested in carefully controlled studies in appropriate animal models. Appropriate laboratory animal studies of interactions between DEET, PB, and permethrin should be conducted.

Finding 13

Reported symptoms suggestive of visceral leishmanial infections include fever, chronic fatigue, malaise, cough, intermittent diarrhea, abdominal pain, weight loss, anemia, lymphadenopathy, and splenomegaly. The committee has considered two aspects of exposure to *L. tropica* and resulting infection with leishmania: the occurrence of either cutaneous or visceral leishmaniasis; and the possibility that some component of the poorly defined illness referred to as "Gulf War Syndrome" may result from leishmania infection.

Leishmaniasis (*L. tropica*) in PGW veterans has been evaluated in some very limited clinical studies, but not in epidemiological studies. The clinical studies suggest that the complex of symptoms in the PGW veterans diagnosed with leishmaniasis differs from what has been described in the literature for other forms of leishmaniasis. A major limitation to further investigation and diagnosis of leishmaniasis is the lack of an informative serologic test or other easy to use screening tests.

Recommendations

- The DoD Joint Technology Coordination Group II has research responsibilities for infectious diseases of military importance and should give high priority to the development of a screening approach to be used under field conditions expected in deployment, and a useful diagnostic test for *L. tropica.* The board also should review the status of leishmania research, with a view toward either drafting a request for proposals for test development, or the structured coordination of existing activities.
- All physicians should be notified to look for symptoms that are consistent with both leishmania infection and those reported as "Gulf War Syndrome." Clear instructions for follow-up actions should be widely communicated throughout the physician community. Veterans of Desert Storm should be notified that if they have symptoms that may suggest viscerotropic leishmaniasis they should bring this possibility to the attention of the staff at any facility where they obtain any health care, whether it is in the VA system or not. The latter may be particularly important due to the potential for long-term survival of leishmania in the host.
- When it becomes feasible, VA, DoD, or both should conduct an epidemiologic and seroepidemiologic study of leishmaniasis in PGW veterans presenting symptoms or conditions and appropriate controls. Special attention should center on a possible relation between leishmaniasis and the "Gulf War Syndrome."

Finding 14

The ecology and epidemiology of *L. tropica* are insufficiently studied. Many important questions remain unanswered concerning host species, vectors, and means of transmission to military personnel. The possible role of dogs as reservoirs of disease and the existence of vectors other than sand flies are questions that have been raised.

Recommendations

- DoD should closely monitor all information regarding ecological and clinical studies of *L. tropica* being conducted in the U.S. and abroad.
- International and U.S. researchers should be queried concerning any advances in diagnostic techniques for identifying *L. tropica.*

Appendix B

Health Consequences of Service During the Persian Gulf War: Recommendations for Research and Information Systems*

CHARGE TO THE COMMITTEE: ITS FINDINGS AND RECOMMENDATIONS

Overview

In this chapter we summarize the findings and principal recommendations of the Committee to Review the Health Consequences of Service During the Persian Gulf War (PGW). Most of the findings are discussed at greater length in the chapters that follow.

Our task was to respond to three specific charges. Each finding is linked to at least one of the charges, and for each we note the principal connection. Recommendations follow each of the findings. The committee was charged as follows.

---

*These findings and recommendations were taken from the Institute of Medicine report, *Health Consequences of Service During the Persian Gulf War: Recommendations for Research and Information Systems,* Washington, D.C.: National Academy Press, 1996.

THE COMMITTEE'S CHARGE

Charge 1

> Assess the effectiveness of actions taken by the Secretary of Veterans Affairs and the Secretary of Defense to collect and maintain information that is potentially useful for assessing the health consequences of military service referred to subsection (a) [of PL 102-585, Persian Gulf (PG) theater of operations during the PGW].

The committee makes four recommendations (recommendations 13–16) in this report regarding the collection and maintenance of information that is potentially useful for assessing the health consequences of military service in the PGW. These recommendations support completion of certain data sets, prompt reporting of research findings and submission for publication in peer-reviewed journals, strengthened medical and epidemiologic research capabilities of the armed forces, and strengthening the decision-making processes for study selection.

Charge 2

> Make recommendations on means of improving the collection and maintenance of such information.

The committee makes five recommendations (recommendations 1, 4, and 8–10) on the collection and maintenance of information on the health consequences of service in the PG. We also give considerable attention to information systems that would be useful in future conflicts. These recommendations are based largely on experience with systems in place for the PGW that have shown some gaps and defects that can be remedied.

Charge 3

> Make recommendations as to whether there is [a] sound scientific basis for an epidemiologic study or studies of the health consequences of such service, and if the recommendation is that there is [a] sound scientific basis for such a study or studies, the nature of the study or studies.

The committee believes that there is indeed a sound basis for epidemiologic studies, and eight recommendations follow (recommendations 2, 3, 5–7, and 11–13).[1] However, the committee does not recommend an additional nationwide epidemiologic study of PG veterans, because such a study is likely to be of limited scientific value at this time. Those large studies that are currently under way should be completed as quickly as possible, while meeting high scientific standards, including a high response rate and a thorough investigation of potential biases, as recommended below.

FINDINGS AND RECOMMENDATIONS

Finding

Recent military deployments, especially in Vietnam and in the Persian Gulf, have demonstrated that concerns about the health consequences of participation in military action may arise long after deployment has ended and that the evaluation of those concerns and the provision of health care to affected personnel may present formidable challenges both to epidemiologists and to medical caregivers. Although some of these challenges can be attributed to the intrinsic difficulty of evaluating poorly understood clusters of events that were not among the expected consequences of combat or of environmental conditions, they also may be attributed in part to limitations of the systems used to collect and manage data regarding the health and service-related exposures of military personnel. No system of record keeping can be expected to provide the information needed to address every unanticipated research issue, including those regarding the health consequences of military service. Nevertheless, the committee has identified several possible improvements in the systems and practices for collecting information on the health and service-related exposures of military personnel. Such changes would increase the ability of the military services to pursue appropriate investigations in the future. Such changes also would increase the capacity of the services to evaluate the efficacy of mobilization-supporting health services (including approaches and methodologies for disease prevention employed before, during, and after mobilization) and would aid in providing the best possible medical care to military service personnel and veterans (Charge 2).

Recommendation 1. The Department of Defense (DoD), the branches of the armed services, and the Department of Veterans Affairs (DVA)

---

[1]Recommendation 13 has been counted as applicable to both Charge 1 and Charge 3, and therefore appears with both.

should continue to work together to develop, fund, and staff medical information systems that include a single, uniform, continuous, and retrievable electronic medical record for each service person. The uniform record should include each relevant health item (including baseline personal risk factors, every inpatient and outpatient medical contact, and all health-related interventions), allow linkage to exposure and other data sets, and have the capability to incorporate relevant medical data from beyond DoD and DVA institutions (e.g., U.S. Public Health Service facilities, civilian medical providers, and other health care institutions). Appropriate consent and protection of individual privacy must be considered for information obtained and included.

Finding

The number and variety of studies regarding consequences of the PGW are already considerable. To date, most health-related studies specifically involving PGW veterans have focused on short-term mental health consequences of deployment, the role of combat exposure, and other stressors experienced in the theater of operations and, to a lesser extent, on problems relating to demobilization and readjustment to civilian life among reservist and National Guard personnel. A few reports have included limited longitudinal follow-up data concerning men and women who served in the PG. Important information may be gained through longer follow-up of some of these groups, particularly since at least one of these groups was first to arrive in the theater, and precombat data are available. Also needed are studies of risk factors in modern deployments predictive of combat stress reactions, posttraumatic stress disorder (PTSD), and other psychiatric disorders of military personnel and veterans. Studies relevant to the trauma of war and the ensuing mental health consequences should concentrate special attention on improving efforts in prevention, intervention, and follow-up (Charge 3).

Recommendation 2. The DoD and DVA should conduct further studies, with appropriate statistical and epidemiological support, to identify risk factors for stress-related psychiatric disorders among military personnel (active and reserve) and to develop better methods to buffer and ameliorate the psychiatric consequences of modern training, deployment, combat, demobilization, and return to daily living.

Recommendation 3. Studies being conducted by DoD and DVA that have included longitudinal follow-up of the mental health of veterans who served in the PG should be supported with continued follow-up after appropriate peer review of study methods. Follow-up in these studies should be sufficient to provide at least a decade of information comparing the mental health status of those deployed with those not deployed.

Finding

The military dominance of U.S. forces in the PGW increased the relative significance of physical and natural environmental exposures as important sources of potential morbidity and mortality, compared with combat injuries. This is likely to recur in future deployments (Charge 2).

Recommendation 4. The DoD should ensure that military medical preparedness for deployments includes detailed attempts to monitor natural and man-made environmental exposures and to prepare for rapid response, early investigation, and accurate data collection, when possible, on physical and natural environmental exposures that are known or possible in the specific theater of operations.

Finding

National Guard and reserve component personnel may differ substantially from active duty personnel in average age, level of training, occupational specialties, family status, and readiness for deployment. Further, it is unclear whether either policies and procedures or the manner in which they are implemented differs between activated reserve or National Guard units and active duty troops for mobilization, deployment, demobilization, and return. All of these factors may affect the health consequences of deployment (Charge 3).

Recommendation 5. Research is needed to determine whether differences in personal characteristics or differences in policies and procedures for mobilization, deployment, demobilization, and return of reserves, National Guard, and regular troops are associated with different or adverse health consequences. If there are associations, strategies necessary to prevent or reduce these adverse health effects should be developed.

Finding

Completed studies have described the mortality experience of troops deployed to the PG during the period of deployment and in the 2-year period after deployment. These studies have documented a consistent pattern of increased risk of death from unintentional injury for the cohort of deployed troops compared with those not deployed to the PG. However, death rates from disease were not significantly increased. Continued monitoring and further study of mortality rates among veterans of the PGW will be of value in assessing the long-term health consequences of deployment (Charge 3).

Recommendation 6. The mortality experience of PG veterans should continue to be monitored for as long as 30 years, on a regular basis, including comparisons with that of PG-era veterans. (PG-era veterans have been defined as those in military service at the time of the PGW, but assigned or deployed elsewhere.) Research investigators should focus on the reported excess mortality from unintentional injury, on mortality from specific illnesses, and on evidence of elevation (or reduction) in the risk of death from other causes.

Recommendation 7. The DVA should exert greater effort to improve understanding of the reasons for excess mortality from unintentional injury. Detailed evaluation is needed beyond death certificate data concerning the circumstances surrounding fatal injury through more focused case-control studies to identify both individual risk factors and remediable causes.

Finding

The armed services and the DVA together are developing a shared basic epidemiological data system, the Defense Medical Epidemiological Database (DMED) (Charge 2).

Recommendation 8. The DMED system should be continued, expanded as planned, expedited to develop the proposed integrated information management system, linked to other key systems, and evaluated regularly.

Finding

Considerable effort has been devoted by DoD to the development of a Troop Exposure Assessment Model (TEAM) for describing the PGW experience of veterans. This has included the completion of an information system designed to establish the geographic location of each unit from January 15, 1991, until the unit departed from the Gulf theater. This system has the potential to be linked to data on regional environmental conditions but will necessarily be devoid of most individual data (such as pesticide exposure or individual health risk factors) (Charge 2).

> **Recommendation 9.** The DoD should complete development of information systems to expeditiously and directly pinpoint unit locations at a high level of disaggregation in space and time (that is, fine detail) and to document local environmental conditions, including appropriate data quality checks, with direct data entry into the system. There is likely to be a need for a similar information system during and after any future conflict, and DoD should prepare and continually update plans for such a nonpaper system. A manual for use of the information systems by research investigators should be compiled, with the strengths and limitations identified.

Finding

The power and complexity of analyses based on space-time geographical information system (GIS) data require careful attention to data quality and the limits imposed by various data items. Quality improvement and assessment of limits are continuous processes and depend on detailed evaluation of data needs for specific analytic questions (Charge 2).

> **Recommendation 10.** For every specific question posed to the current TEAM, DoD should assess the strengths and limitations of the TEAM as a resource for evaluating the health significance of geographically defined exposures of troops, including those in the PGW and those in conflicts that may develop in the future. Evaluations and recommendations for possible modification of the TEAM should be reported to the PG Coordinating Board, Research Working Group.

Finding

Given the unprecedented numbers of women serving in the PG, especially those in largely new roles, including combat support, it is important to specially evaluate the health consequences and needs for health services of women who served in the PG. Preliminary findings from studies being conducted at the Boston VA Medical Center (VAMC) indicate that additional research in this area is needed. Additional research is also needed on the health effects of having male and female personnel serve together in combat or under threat of combat (Charge 3).

> **Recommendation 11.** The DoD and DVA should ensure that studies of the health effects of deployment, including effects on PGW veterans, include evaluation of exposures, experiences, and situations of both women and men, with attention to their age, prior military service, marital and parental status, and other gender-specific parameters.
>
> **Recommendation 12.** The DoD and DVA should conduct studies of the health consequences of assigning men and women to serve together in combat or under the threat of enemy action. Such work should be undertaken with a focus on prevention and amelioration of any added stresses.

Finding

Several important studies are currently under way. Worthwhile data are being collected and prepared, and the studies should be completed promptly, with the necessary personnel and funding to collect the additional data needed, to conduct appropriate analyses, and to evaluate potential biases. Findings from these studies are likely to provide leads as to whether or not additional research along these lines is required to produce more specific findings (Charges 1 and 3).

• The Naval Health Research Center at San Diego has undertaken a series of studies under the general title of "Epidemiologic Studies of Morbidity Among Gulf War Veterans: A Search for Etiologic Agents and Risk Factors." These studies hold promise for answering some important questions about the health of PGW veterans after demobilization and about the possibility that veterans and their spouses may experience an excess risk of adverse pregnancy outcomes as a result of service in the PGW. The studies are being carried out with care, excellent planning, and proper pilot efforts to determine feasibility.

Upon completion, these studies should provide important guidance concerning whether veterans have experienced hospitalization at rates in excess of their nondeployed peers, have developed specific symptoms or illnesses related to their PGW experience, or have experienced risks that have resulted in adverse reproductive outcomes related to their service in the Gulf.

> **Recommendation 13a.** The Naval Health Research studies in San Diego should be completed and results published as designed and scheduled.

• Although there are significant problems with the DVA National Health Survey, the investigators have designed additional phases of the study that will be important to complete. The physical examinations and follow-up of nonrespondents to the mail survey will be an important step toward describing potential biases and evaluating signs and symptoms of both PG and PG-era study participants.

> **Recommendation 13b.** The DVA National Health Survey should be completed and results published as designed and scheduled.

• The DVA-DoD study that was designed to examine predictors of enrollment in the DVA PG Health Registry (PGHR) may provide useful information as to what objectively measurable factors contribute to self-selection into the registry. In addition to the proposed analysis of associations among demographics, past health experiences, and health behaviors as possible predictors of enrollment, information on the eligibility of individuals for health care, as well as the type of health care, could generate additional hypotheses to be investigated.

> **Recommendation 13c.** Evaluation of predictors of enrollment in the DVA PGHR should be promptly completed and results published. Included, if possible, should be information on type of care requested, required, and received.

Finding

The armed forces have had small but high-quality and effective capabilities in epidemiology. Recent cutbacks have reduced these capabilities, with potentially serious effects on both military preparedness and the health care of veterans. The Theater Area Medical Laboratory (TAML) is an example of how specialists can respond rapidly to potential health problems of troops deployed in various areas of the world and provide immediate and useful information necessary to maintain the military readiness of the armed forces. In addition, well-trained epidemiologists and preventive medicine specialists are necessary for conducting the relevant population-based epidemiologic studies, with comprehensive exposure assessment, that have the greatest likelihood of being informative about the health consequences of any future deployment. Such capability should permit studies that extend beyond the time of an individual's active duty service and that are capable of responding to questions of delayed effects that may emerge only years, or even decades, after a military operation (Charge 1).

> **Recommendation 14.** The epidemiologic capabilities of the armed forces should be strengthened rather than reduced. The command structure should be kept informed about the reasons for and the results of this recommendation and its relevance to military preparedness and effectiveness, and should be encouraged to support appropriate epidemiologic work in the theater of operations and in the postdeployment period.

Finding

Much good work on symptom complexes and other matters discussed in this report has been done by DoD, DVA, and their contractors. However, it is evident from the references cited in this report that many are in the "gray literature"—available to those who know they exist and how to ask for them, but not published in the open, peer-reviewed scientific literature where they will be fully indexed and readily available, with some assurance that they meet at least minimal scientific standards. Even this committee, with the contacts and expertise it developed over time, had difficulty in identifying and obtaining some of these reports. The committee also is concerned about the high cost of much recent research and the necessity for maximizing the nation's overall return on that investment. In summary, the committee believes that health-related research is not finalized until it is published and readily accessible in peer-reviewed journals (Charge 1).

> **Recommendation 15.** The DoD and DVA should adopt a policy that internal and contract-supported reports on health research will be submitted for publication in the peer-reviewed scientific literature in a timely manner.

Finding

Some research directed toward reports of unexplained illnesses after the PGW was flawed in the questions posed, populations studied, or research design. We believe that these defects could have been identified before research projects were funded if requests for proposals had been announced generally and had been open to the scientific community at large and if fully developed research proposals had been reviewed by panels of qualified expert peers. Some research was announced and reviewed in this manner, but much more could be so treated, to the benefit of both veterans and the public (Charge 1).

> **Recommendation 16.** The Congress, DVA, and DoD should adopt a policy that unless there are well-specified, openly stated reasons to the contrary, requests for proposals for research related to unexplained illnesses or other needed health-related research will be publicly announced and open to the scientific community at large, that proposals will be reviewed by panels of appropriately qualified experts, and that funding will follow the recommendations of those experts.

Appendix C

Evaluation of the U.S. Department of Defense Persian Gulf Comprehensive Clinical Evaluation Program: Overall Assessment and Recommendations*

1.) OVERALL ASSESSMENT OF THE CCEP GOALS PROCEDURES:

The Comprehensive Clinical Evaluation Program (CCEP) clinical protocol is a thorough, systematic approach to the diagnosis of a wide spectrum of diseases. A specific medical diagnosis or diagnoses can be reached for most patients by using the CCEP protocol. The Department of Defense (DoD) has made conscientious efforts to build consistency and quality assurance into this program at the many medical treatment facilities (MTFs) and regional medical centers (RMCs) across the country.

The committee is impressed with the quality of the design and the efficiency of the implementation of the clinical protocol, the considerable devotion of resources to this program, and the remarkable amount of work that has been accomplished in a year. The high professional standards, commitment, and diligence of the physicians involved in the CCEP at the RMCs were readily apparent at the three committee meetings. The committee commends the DoD for its efforts to provide high-quality medical care in the CCEP and the success that it has achieved to date in developing the infrastructure necessary to efficiently contact, schedule, refer, and track thousands of patients through the system.

---

*This appendix is excerpted from the Institute of Medicine report, *Evaluation of the U.S. Department of Defense Persian Gulf Comprehensive Clinical Evaluation,* Washington, D.C.: National Academy Press, 1996.

Overall, the systematic, comprehensive set of clinical practice guidelines set forth in the CCEP are appropriate, and they have assisted physicians in the determination of specific diagnoses for thousands of patients across the country.

2.) GENERAL RECOMMENDATIONS FOR THE IMPLEMENTATION OF THE CCEP:

2.1.) Referrals of Patients from Phase I to Phase II of the CCEP:

2.1.1.) Structure and revise the CCEP protocol and logistics to allow the majority of patients to receive a final diagnosis by Phase I:

Currently, the majority of patients do not receive a final diagnosis until Phase II, yet some of these patients have straightforward medical problems. The Committee recommends that final diagnoses could be reached in Phase I if more diagnostic resources are made available. This major change would require the availability of substantial numbers of internists or family practitioners at MTFs to perform comprehensive evaluations. It would also require better, more consistent explanations to MTF physicians about the purposes and procedures of the CCEP. It would require regional medical center physicians to provide adequate quality assurance of MTF work-ups and timely feedback to MTF providers.

On January 17, 1995, the DoD adopted these suggestions by setting goals that about 80% of patients would receive a definitive diagnosis at an MTF level. For some patients, this change has required specialty consultations at the MTF, as well as advice from an RMC physician. These changes necessitated an enhanced quality control role by the RMC physician and prompt, appropriate feedback to the MTF physician.

2.1.2.) Curtail diagnostic work-ups in patients not seriously disabled with minor complaints:

Initially, patients who do not accept their initial diagnosis could request a continued evaluation all the way through Phase II. The Committee recommends that diagnostic work-ups in patients not seriously disabled but with minor complaints should be curtailed. Alternatively, if a physician has made a definitive diagnosis and appropriate treatment has been given, the evaluation would be concluded. On January 17, 1995, the DoD implemented the suggestions that referral to Phase II be made on the basis of the clinical judgment of the primary care physician, and patients were no longer permitted to self-refer to an RMC.

2.1.3.) Require additional efforts to provide more care at the primary care level:

The Committee encourages efforts to provide more care at the primary care level, because they will enhance the continuity of care and will foster the establishment of an ongoing therapeutic relationship.

2.1.4.) Continue referral of subgroups of patients whose illnesses are difficult to diagnose:

Patients whose illnesses are difficult to diagnose should continue to be referred to Phase II at an RMC. The decision to refer to Phase II should be based on the clinical judgment of the primary care physician, which, in turn, would be dependent on the clarity of the patient's diagnoses and the feasibility of the proposed treatment program at the MTF level. The DoD should continue its goal of enhanced accessibility of RMC physicians to allow regular consultations with MTF primary care physicians on patients with more complex diagnoses.

2.2.) Systematic Guidelines for Psychiatric Referrals and Adequacy of Psychiatric Resources:

2.2.1.) Develop explicit guidelines for the identification of Phase I patients who would benefit from a psychiatric evaluation:

CCEP physicians have noted the need for standardized guidelines for screening, assessing, evaluating, and treating patients. Such Phase I guidelines should be developed to help ensure adequate psychiatric resources for both the initial evaluation and long-term follow-up care.

2.2.2.) Alert primary care physicians about the high prevalence of psychiatric disorders:

Two methods that have been proposed by RMC physicians to expedite the scheduling of psychiatric evaluations would be (1) the more frequent use of civilian psychiatrists and (2) consideration of using Ph.D.-level psychologists, as well as psychiatrists, when necessary.

3.) SPECIFIC OBSERVATIONS OF AND RECOMMENDATIONS FOR THE IMPLEMENTATION OF THE CCEP:

3.1.) Analysis and Interpretation of the CCEP Results:

3.1.1.) Symptoms and diagnoses in the CCEP population:

3.1.1.1.) No evidence has been found that the DoD has been trying to avoid reaching a single unifying diagnosis:

The committee found no evidence that the DoD has been trying to avoid reaching a single "unifying" diagnosis when a plausible one was available. A "unifying" diagnosis is defined here as a single diagnosis that could explain most or all of a patient's symptoms.

3.1.1.2.) Signs and symptoms in many patients can be explained by well-recognized conditions:

One interpretation of the CCEP results is that the signs and symptoms in many patients can be explained by well-recognized conditions that are readily diagnosable and treatable. The committee concludes that this is a more likely interpretation than the interpretation that a high proportion of the CCEP patients are suffering from a unique, previously unknown "mystery disease."

3.1.1.3.) Provide more detailed information on specific diagnoses in future reports:

By providing more detailed information on specific diagnoses in its future reports, the DoD might help correct the impressions among the general public that exist about the high degree of prevalence of a "mystery disease" or a new, unique "Persian Gulf Syndrome."

3.1.1.4.) Investigate the diagnosis in patients with disability processing actions:

Disability processing actions in the Services' Physical Disability Processing Systems have been completed for 246 of the 10,020 CCEP patients. The DoD has not provided any data about their diagnoses or their reasons for medical separation from the military. The committee recommends that the DoD investigate the diagnoses in this group of patients in future reports, as well as whether or not the disorders could have been caused or exacerbated by service in the Persian Gulf.

3.1.1.5.) Don't view CCEP results as estimates of the prevalence of disability related to Persian Gulf service:

Many other individuals who served in the Persian Gulf have left active service and, hence, are not eligible for the DoD's CCEP. Some of these veterans may have disabilities related or unrelated to their service in the Persian Gulf, and those with disabilities might be more likely to have left active service. For these reasons, the CCEP results should not be viewed as estimates of the prevalence of disability related to Persian Gulf service.

3.1.2.) Evidence of a New, Unique Persian Gulf Syndrome:

3.1.2.1.) There is a lack of clinical evidence of a unique Persian Gulf Syndrome:

The committee agrees with DoD that there is currently no clinical evidence in the CCEP of a previously unknown, serious illness among Persian Gulf veterans. If there were a new or unique illness or syndrome among Persian Gulf veterans that could cause serious impairment in a high proportion of veterans at risk, it would probably be detectable in the population of 10,020 CCEP patients. On the other hand, if an unknown illness were mild or affected only a small proportion of veterans at risk, it might not be detectable in a case series, no matter how large.

3.1.2.2.) Share the entire CCEP data set with qualified researchers outside of the DoD:

The committee encourages the DoD's plan to share the entire CCEP data set with qualified researchers outside of the DoD who might be able to undertake the kind of research with the methodological sophistication that the identification of a new syndrome would require.

3.1.3.) Potential Relationship of Illnesses in CCEP Patients to Service in the Persian Gulf:

3.1.3.1.) Discuss the issue of causality explicitly and unambiguously in its future reports:

Physicians involved with the development and the administration of the CCEP have, in various public presentations, acknowledged that some CCEP patients have developed illnesses that are directly related to their service in the Persian Gulf. The recent DoD report on 10,020 CCEP participants, however, only touches on this issue indirectly. The committee encourages the DoD to discuss the issue of causality explicitly and unambiguously in its future reports. Such a discussion might help to alleviate the current climate of confusion and mistrust that exists among some Persian Gulf veterans and the general public.

3.1.3.2.) Determine the timing of the onset of disease:

The committee recommends that the DoD attempt to determine the timing of the onset of disease, especially for patients who have significant impairments. Review of military or civilian medical records that predate enrollment in the CCEP may provide contemporaneous documentation of the onset of symptoms in some patients, especially if the symptoms are serious. In addition, it is important to determine whether service in the Persian Gulf has contributed to the exacerbation of preexisting diseases in some CCEP patients.

3.1.4.) Comparison of the CCEP Population with Other Populations:

3.1.4.1.) Be cautious about comparison with other populations:

In its most recent report, the DoD compares the symptoms and diagnoses in the CCEP population with the symptoms and diagnoses in several community-based and clinically based populations. In the committee's view, interpretations based on comparisons with other populations should be made with great caution and only with the explicit recognition of the limitations of the CCEP as a self-selected case series. The CCEP was not designed to answer epidemiological questions, such as how the frequencies of certain diagnoses compare between the CCEP population and a control population. Instead, it was designed as a medical evaluation and treatment program. Indeed, the research aims of the CCEP do not appear to be stated explicitly, nor does there appear to be a concrete epidemiological study plan. Without research hypotheses, it is not possible to judge whether any particular comparison group is appropriate. Each individual population should be described to prevent confusion.

3.1.4.2.) It's difficult to establish causal relationships by relying on CCEP data alone:

It would be extremely difficult to establish causal relationships or to identify and characterize a new "Persian Gulf Syndrome" definitively by relying on data from the CCEP alone. The latitude permitted in the clinical examination program conflicts with the rigor necessary to answer an epidemiological question.

3.1.4.3.) Consider the CCEP data to have high clinical utility:

The CCEP data do have considerable clinical utility, and they could be used to address many important questions from a descriptive perspective. Many case series could be derived from these data. In addition, the results of the clinical exams could provide guidance in the selection of research questions and in the design of future epidemiological research. The CCEP findings could be used to generate epidemiological questions on other types of diseases that are much more frequent in the CCEP population, such as musculoskeletal diseases.

3.2.) Specific Medical Diagnosis:

3.2.1.) Psychiatric Conditions:

3.2.1.1.) Make patients aware of psychiatric conditions and their prevalence and morbidity:

Patients need to understand that psychiatric conditions and disorders are real diseases that cause real symptoms and that diagnoses are made with objective criteria and are not merely "labels" applied because physical abnormalities were not found. The CCEP patients, as well as their primary care physicians, also need to understand the prevalence of and the concomitant morbidity that result from psychiatric disorders in the general population (major depression, for example). Finally, the CCEP patients need to be aware that effective treatments that actually ameliorate symptoms exist for many of these disorders.

3.2.1.2.) Emphasize effects and diagnosis of psychosocial stressors:

In its future reports, the DoD is encouraged to emphasize that psychosocial stressors can produce physical and psychological effects that are as real and potentially devastating as physical, chemical, or biological stressors. The DoD should also emphasize that thorough efforts to diagnose psychiatric conditions in the CCEP population may lead to appropriate, successful treatments.

3.2.1.3.) Identify people with risk of developing depression or Post-Traumatic Stress Disorder (PTSD):

The committee is particularly concerned about the CCEP patients who have developed or who are at risk of developing major depression or PTSD. These people need to be identified and provided with some form of preventive intervention.

3.2.1.4.) Improve standardization of psychiatric evaluations:

The committee recommends that the DoD consider methods of improving the standardization of the psychiatric evaluations in the CCEP. The DoD should consider establishing detailed guidelines for the psychiatric evaluations and should attempt to obtain greater standardization of these evaluations among the various hospitals across the country. These guidelines could provide suggested procedures for the use of selected self-report instruments for the assessment of the most commonly diagnosed disorders, as well as procedures for more in-depth structured clinical interviews when indicated.

3.2.1.5.) Document and investigate the onset and course of symptoms and psychosocial stressors:

It would be especially important to document the onset and course of symptoms and to investigate their possible link with psychosocial stressors associated with mobilization and return home, as well as with service-related exposures in the Persian Gulf region. This assessment would require an additional set of questions to supplement the questionnaire currently used in Phase I of the CCEP. The thorough assessment of psychosocial stressors is essential information for treatment planning for patients with complex, chronic symptoms.

3.2.1.6.) Standardize neuropsychological evaluations:

Standardization of the neuropsychological evaluations is a related concern. The neuropsychological methods vary from pencil and paper testing at some sites to computer-administered testing at other sites. One method of achieving a better consensus is to convene a meeting attended by one psychiatrist and one neuropsychologist from each center to attempt to standardize their methods.

3.2.1.7.) Standardize classification and coding of diseases:

In addition to the standardization of psychiatric evaluations in the CCEP, the classification and coding of these diseases should also be standardized.

3.2.1.8.) Document headache categories differently:

The classification of different types of headaches into three separate categories may be consistent with ICD-9 coding rules, but the DoD should also report a special tabulation that combines all headaches into one group.

3.2.1.9.) Add explicit written instruction on medical record-keeping and coding:

More explicit written instructions could be added to the CCEP guidelines to help prevent the most frequent problems found in the medical record-keeping and coding. Committee comments about inconsistencies are mainly aimed at the quality control necessary for accurate reporting of summary data rather than at the quality of the medical care itself.

3.2.1.10.) Expand discussion of psychological stressors:

DoD should consider expanding discussion of the psychological stressors that were present during the Persian Gulf War.

3.2.1.11.) Utilize results of on-going studies to revise CCEP:

It is possible that the DoD will be able to use the results of on-going epidemiologic studies on psychiatric conditions to revise the CCEP, that is, to revise the standardized questionnaires or to add or delete targeted lab tests or specialty consultations. In addition, the CCEP clinicians may be able to utilize these results in the counseling and treatment of their patients. These results may also be useful for the DoD in its planning to minimize the effects of psychosocial stressors in future deployments through the use of preventive medicine interventions.

3.2.2.) Musculoskeletal Conditions:

3.2.2.1.) Provide more details of diagnostic categorization of musculoskeletal conditions:

The draft and final DoD reports on 10,020 CCEP patients do not provide adequate details for the IOM committee to make a thorough evaluation of the diagnostic categorization of musculoskeletal conditions. More explanation about the diagnostic aspects of these musculoskeletal conditions would be useful, for example, information on single-joint involvement versus multijoint conditions or articular versus non-articular conditions. In addition, details on disease severity and disease activity would be useful.

3.2.2.2.) Place more emphasis on musculoskeletal conditions:

The DoD and the DVA should consider placing more emphasis on research on musculoskeletal conditions, since these are the most prevalent disorders among the CCEP populations.

3.2.3.) Signs, Symptoms, and Ill-Defined Conditions:

3.2.3.1.) Clarify types of disorders included in the ICD-9 category:

The committee recommends that in future reports the DoD attempt to clarify the types of disorders that are included in the ICD-9 category of signs, symptoms, and ill-defined conditions (SSIDC). Individuals with these signs, symptoms, and ill-defined conditions should be evaluated in a rigorous manner, just as individuals with any other symptoms are evaluated.

3.2.4.) Infectious Diseases:

3.2.4.1.) Infectious disease is not a frequent cause of serious illness:

The IOM committee concludes that infectious diseases are not a frequent cause of serious illness in the CCEP population.

3.2.4.2.) Veterans are not likely afflicted with some previously unknown pathogen:

On the basis of the current evidence, it is unlikely that a significant proportion of Persian Gulf veterans are afflicted with some previously unknown pathogen that is evading the current diagnostic efforts.

3.2.5.) Chronic Fatigue Syndrome, Fibromyalgia, and Multiple Chemical Sensitivity:

3.2.5.1.) Estimating prevalence of chronic fatigue syndrome, fibromyalgia, and multiple chemical sensitivity is difficult:

The IOM committee's review of the CCEP protocol suggests that data on chronic fatigue syndrome (CFS), fibromyalgia (FM), and multiple chemical sensitivity (MCS) may have been collected by various diagnostic methods. For this reason, it is not possible to estimate the prevalence of these conditions from the CCEP data.

3.2.5.2.) Collect data using established diagnostic criteria for CFS and FM:

In the clinical evaluations, data should be collected by using established diagnostic criteria for CFS and FM.

3.2.5.3.) Established diagnostic criteria do not exist for MCS:

A widely accepted set of diagnostic criteria does not exist for MCS. Consequently, the medical evaluation in CCEP cannot be expected to diagnose the clinical syndrome of MCS.

3.2.5.4.) Include CFS, FM, and MCS in on-going and future epidemiological research studies:

If more is to be learned about the relationship between these disorders (CFS, FM, and MCS) and Persian Gulf service, they should be included among the epidemiological research studies that are ongoing or planned for the future.

3.2.5.5.) Continue thorough workup to diagnose sleep disturbances and fatigue:

Because of the thorough, systematic workup mandated in the CCEP, many disorders that could contribute to sleep disturbance and fatigue have been diagnosed. These diligent efforts to unmask occult medical problems that could substantially contribute to fatigue have been productive and should continue.

3.3.) Use of the CCEP Results for Education Improvements in the Medical Protocol and Outcome Evaluations:

3.3.1.) Use of the CCEP Results for Education:

3.3.1.1.) Continue public release of analysis results of the CCEP on an on-going, periodic basis:

The IOM committee encourages the DoD to continue to release its analysis of the results of the CCEP on an ongoing, periodic basis. Several audiences that would be interested in these results include active-duty members of the service, veterans, members of the U.S. Congress, the lay media, as well as military, DVA, and civilian medical and public health professionals. The CCEP medical findings would also be of interest to physicians in the DVA system and in the general community.

3.3.1.2.) Distribute CCEP findings to all primary care physicians at MTFs and RMCs:

The medical findings of the CCEP should be distributed promptly to all primary care physicians at the MTFs and RMCs. This would provide feedback on their diagnostic decision-making. Information on the frequencies of particular symptoms and their specific diagnoses made in the CCEP population could be useful, for instance, in developing a differential diagnosis for individual patients.

3.3.1.3.) Develop a more concise version of the DoD report for active-duty service personnel and veterans:

A more concise version of the DoD report on 10,020 patients, written in nontechnical language and with clearly stated conclusions, should be developed for a target audience of active-duty service personnel and veterans. If the DoD developed and distributed a fact sheet or newsletter aimed at Persian Gulf veterans, the information on the CCEP would be more accurate and more comprehensive than most reports in the general news media. This would also provide an additional opportunity to notify the readers about the availability of the medical exam in the CCEP, the hotline number, and the eligibility criteria.

3.3.1.4.) Develop a more comprehensive document describing potential exposures in more detail:

The DoD should also consider developing for clinical use in the CCEP a more comprehensive document that describes the many potential exposures in more detail. Any document that is prepared, however, must make clear what is known and what is unknown about the relationship between these stressors and the physical or psychological consequences.

3.3.2.) Use of the CCEP Results to Improve the Medical Protocol:

3.3.2.1.) Use CCEP examination results to improve standardization practices:

The DoD now has results on the examinations of more than 10,000 CCEP patients, which could be used to improve the standardized questionnaires, lab tests, and specialty consultations.

3.3.2.2.) Refine questions related to potential psychological stressors:

More refined questions related to potential psychological stressors could be added systematically to the Phase I medical history. The CCEP physicians might find this information useful in diagnosing and counseling their patients. In addition, it may be possible to identify patients who are at increased risk of psychological problems on the basis of their experiences in the war. Perhaps explicit questions on death exposure and other known risk factors could be added to the Phase I questionnaire.

3.3.2.3.) Determine if lab tests or specialty consultations should be added to Phase I:

The CCEP results should be analyzed to determine whether there are lab tests or specialty consultations that should be added systematically to Phase I to increase its diagnostic yield. Diseases that are diagnosed relatively frequently in Phase II may often be overlooked in Phase I. If such diseases could be identified, perhaps appropriate screening instruments could be added to Phase I.

3.3.2.4.) Compare and coordinate methods and clinical results of the CCEP and UCAP:

The DVA uses a protocol similar to that used in the CCEP called the Uniform Case Assessment Protocol (UCAP). The methods and clinical results of the CCEP and UCAP should be compared to coordinate and improve the two programs.

3.3.3.) Use of the CCEP Results for Patient Outcome:

3.3.3.1.) Perform targeted patient evaluations:

On the basis of more than 10,000 patient evaluations to date, RMC physicians could begin to perform a series of targeted patient evaluations. The most common diseases in the CCEP could be identified, and suggested approaches to patient treatment could be developed. Consensus guidelines for the treatment and counseling of CCEP patients who have the most common disorders could be useful for primary care physicians.

3.3.3.2.) Communicate successful treatment methods between RMCs:

If one RMC has had a lot of experience with a particular disease category and some measure of success in its treatment, the DoD could ensure that a description of their successful methods is communicated to the other MTFs and RMCs across the country.

3.3.3.3.) Review disorders among CCEP patients who have applied for disability payments or for medical discharge from the service:

The DoD could perform a review of the types and severities of the disorders among CCEP patients who have applied for disability payments or for medical discharge from the service. In addition, the final disposition of these cases could be evaluated, including the potential relationship between particular diseases and Persian Gulf service. The DoD could use the results of these disability determinations to predict which diseases are likely to be associated with the most impairment among CCEP patients in the future. The DoD could also use these results to develop rehabilitation and early intervention methods for impaired Persian Gulf veterans, such as the Specialized Care Centers (SCC). Another reason to analyze these disability claims would be to investigate possible preexisting risk factors for the development of the impairment. If such risk factors are identifiable, then targeted preventive medicine interventions could be planned for individuals participating in future overseas deployments.

3.3.4.) Specialized Care Center (SCC):

3.3.4.1.) The DoD has made serious efforts to develop an SCC program that has ambitious goals:

The IOM committee concludes that the DoD has made serious efforts to develop an SCC program with ambitious goals for a select group of seriously impaired military personnel. The committee's review should be considered preliminary, however, because it is based on one visit and it is still early in the development of the program.

3.3.4.2.) Provide multidisciplinary treatment modalities:

The SCC currently performs a thorough reevaluation of each patient's medical problems. SCC physicians should consider limiting the diagnostic role that they play to focusing on the incoming patients who have been very difficult to diagnose at the RMC level. Instead, the SCC should focus on providing multidisciplinary treatment modalities that are not readily available at the RMC level.

3.3.4.3.) Need for individualized follow-up and therapeutic regimens:

The need for individualized follow-up is crucial for the types of difficult patients who are likely to be treated at the SCC. Medical staff at the SCC will need to know whether a particular therapeutic plan is feasible at the patient's nearest MTF and whether long-term follow-up care can be performed. The primary care physician at the MTF needs to encourage continuous patient compliance with the carefully designed, individualized therapeutic regimens.

3.3.4.4.) Develop objective measure of functional status for follow-up evaluation:

The SCC physicians should develop a set of relatively objective measures of functional status for the follow-up evaluation. These could include (1) appropriate utilization of medical care, (2) appropriate use of medications or other methods to cope with symptoms, (3) general level of activities of daily living, (4) employment status, and (5) status of interpersonal relationships.

3.3.4.5.) Evaluate the SCC program itself:

The SCC program itself needs an evaluation component after several of its graduates have returned for their 6-month reevaluations. Several issues will need to be evaluated in light of the successes and barriers that the program has experienced, including eligibility criteria for patients; roles of the SCC in a diagnostic reevaluation of patients; successful continuity of care of patients, with shared responsibility by the SCC and MTFs; and the unique need for the SCC, beyond the usual standard of a tertiary care medical center.

3.3.4.6.) DoD has taken a serious approach to the treatment and rehabilitation of these patients in the SCC:

The committee believes that the DoD has taken a serious approach to the treatment and rehabilitation of these impaired patients who have treatable, chronic diseases.

3.3.4.7.) Investigate costs and benefits of the SCC program:

Because this program is very labor-intensive, it is probably very expensive on a per-patient basis. At the same time, the potential benefits for each patient could be high, if successful rehabilitation of serious, long-term impairment can be achieved. Subsequent evaluations of the SCC program should investigate its costs and benefits, if possible.

3.3.4.8.) Identify the most effective elements of the SCC program:

If the SCC program is successful in improving the health and functional status of its patients, perhaps the elements that are most effective in enabling the patients to cope with their symptoms could be identified. Perhaps some of these elements could be disseminated and integrated into existing MTF programs that are close to where CCEP patients live and work.

3.4.) Research Relevant to the CCEP:

3.4.1.) Epidemiological Research Relevant to the CCEP:

3.4.1.1.) Utilize on-going epidemiological studies for revising or improving the CCEP:

The results of on-going epidemiological studies may be useful for making revisions or improvements in the CCEP medical protocol itself, for example, to revise the standardized questionnaires or to add or delete targeted lab tests. The study results may also be useful in the counseling and treatment of CCEP patients.

3.4.1.2.) Acknowledge the serious limitations of the CCEP data for epidemiological purposes:

Data from individuals in the CCEP are also being used in some of these epidemiological studies. In these studies, the serious limitations of the CCEP data for epidemiological purposes that were previously identified must be kept in mind.

3.4.2.) Exposure Assessment Research Relevant to the CCEP:

3.4.2.1.) Investigate experiences of individuals in UICs with higher rates of CCEP participation:

The IOM committee encourages DoD to perform further investigations on the war and postwar experiences of individuals in the Unit Identification Codes (UICs) with higher rates of CCEP participation.

3.4.2.2.) Investigate exposures restricted to particular locations or special occupational groups:

The committee encourages the DoD to investigate exposures that were restricted to particular locations or special occupational groups, such as troops who had direct combat exposure. The types of symptoms and diseases in CCEP participants in these special groups and UICs could be analyzed and contrasted with the symptoms and diagnoses of CCEP participants in other units.

COMMITTEE ON THE DOD PERSIAN GULF SYNDROME COMPREHENSIVE CLINICAL EVALUATION PROGRAM

Gerard Burrow,* *Chair*, Dean, Yale University School of Medicine, New Haven, Connecticut

Dan Blazer,* Dean of Medical Education and Professor of Psychiatry, Duke University Medical Center, Durham, North Carolina

Margit Bleecker, Director, Center for Occupational and Environmental Neurology, Baltimore, Maryland

*Member, Institute of Medicine.

Ralph Horwitz, Chairman, Department of Internal Medicine, Yale University School of Medicine, New Haven, Connecticut

Howard Kipen, Associate Professor and Director, Occupational Health Division, Robert Wood Johnson Medical School, Piscataway, New Jersey

Adel Mahmoud,* Chairman, Department of Medicine, Case Western Reserve University and University Hospitals of Cleveland, Cleveland, Ohio

Michael Osterholm, State Epidemiologist, Minnesota Department of Health, Minneapolis, Minnesota

Robert Pynoos, Professor of Psychiatry, University of California at Los Angeles, Los Angeles, California

Anthony Scialli, Associate Professor, Department of Obstetrics and Gynecology, Georgetown University Medical Center, Washington, D.C.

Rosemary Sokas, Associate Professor of Medicine, Division of Occupational and Environmental Medicine, George Washington University School of Medicine, Washington, D.C.

Guthrie Turner, Chief Medical Consultant, Division of Disability Determination Services, State of Washington, Tummwater, Washington

Michael Weisman, Professor, Division of Rheumatology, University of California at San Diego Medical Center, San Diego, California

Staff

Michael A. Stoto, Director, Division of Health Promotion and Disease Prevention

Kelley A. Brix, Study Director

Deborah Katz, Research Assistant

Amy Noel O'Hara, Project Assistant

Donna D. Thompson, Division Assistant

Mona Brinegar, Financial Associate

Appendix D

Adequacy of the Comprehensive Clinical Evaluation Program: Nerve Agents*

RECOMMENDATIONS

The charge to the committee was to determine whether the Comprehensive Clinical Evaluation Program could adequately diagnose and treat possible health problems among service personnel who may have been exposed to low levels of nerve agents. The committee reviewed extensive clinical and research results regarding the effects of nerve agents. No evidence available to the committee conclusively indicated the existence of long-term health effects of low-level exposure to nerve agents. Because firm conclusions about these effects remain elusive, the committee reviewed information about the types of health effects that *might* exist as a result of exposure. Leading scientists presented information suggesting that the possible effects *might* include neurological problems such as peripheral sensory neuropathies and psychiatric problems such as alterations in mood, cognition, or behavior.

Recent reports suggesting a possible toxic synergistic effect following exposure to multiple agents known to influence cholinesterase activity will require extensive research to determine their significance (Haley and Kurt, 1997; Haley et al., 1997a,b; Lottie et al., 1993). The results of the research to date, however, did not appear to indicate any additional possible health effects should be considered by the committee other than those already identified.

---

*This appendix is excerpted from the Institute of Medicine report, *Adequacy of the Comprehensive Clinical Evaluation Program: Nerve Agents,* Washington, D.C.: National Academy Press, 1997.

The committee concluded that the CCEP continues to provide an appropriate screening approach to the diagnosis of disease. Most CCEP patients receive a diagnosis and 80% of participants receive more than one diagnosis. Although the types of primary diagnoses commonly seen in the CCEP involve a variety of conditions, 65% of all primary diagnoses fall into three diagnostic groups (1) psychological conditions; (2) musculoskeletal diseases; and (3) symptoms, signs, ill-defined conditions or a fourth group designated as "healthy." **However, in view of potential exposure to low levels of nerve agents, certain refinements in the CCEP would increase its value.** These refinements are viewed as part of a natural evolution and improvement process and, therefore, need not be applied retrospectively. The committee does encourage rapid implementation in order to provide the benefits of an improved system to new enrollees.

The committee recommends improved documentation of the screening used during Phase I for patients with psychological conditions such as depression and posttraumatic stress disorder (PTSD). The DoD (DoD, 1996) reported that depression and PTSD account for a substantial percentage of those receiving a diagnosis of a psychological condition. In addition, if there are long-term health effects of nerve agent exposure, it is possible that these effects could be manifested as changes in mood or behavior. The committee will be conducting an in-depth examination of the adequacy of the CCEP as it relates to stress and psychiatric disorders at a later time; however, because of the increased importance of ensuring that all possibilities are thoroughly checked, better documentation in this area is encouraged. Primary physicians could use any of a number of self-report screening scales, but consistent use of the same scale across facilities would ensure consistent results.

The committee recommends improved documentation of neurological screening done during both Phase I and Phase II of the CCEP. Concern about nerve agent exposure as well as the number of nonspecific, undiagnosed illnesses among CCEP patients makes documentation of neurological screening extremely important. CCEP patients are referred to neuromuscular specialists if they have complaints of severe muscle weakness, fatigue, or myalgias lasting for at least 6 months that significantly interfere with activities of daily living. These patients are evaluated by board-certified neurologists who have subspecialty training in neuromuscular disease. Based on the description of the tests administered and examinations conducted, the committee finds that the CCEP is sufficient to ensure that no chronic, well-established neurological problem is being overlooked. The documentation of the use of these tests and procedures, however, could and should be improved. Such improvements would engender confidence that neurological examinations and treatments across facilities are comparable.

Given the importance of thorough neurological and psychiatric screening, **the committee recommends that Phase I primary physicians have ready access to a referral neurologist and a referral psychiatrist.** As mentioned earlier, patients are referred to neuromuscular specialists if they have complaints of severe muscle weakness, fatigue, or myalgias lasting for at least 6 months that significantly interfere with activities of daily living. Appropriate psychiatric referrals could include those with chronic depression that is treatment-resistant, an unexplained, persistent complaint of memory problems, or significant impairment secondary to behavioral difficulties, such as not being able to maintain productive work due to behavioral abnormalities. While patients referred for Phase II consultations with a neurologist or psychiatrist are cared for adequately, it is sometimes difficult for the primary physician to determine whether or not a referral is appropriate. In such instances, the physician tends to refer more frequently than not. It may be that, if the primary care physician had neurological and psychiatric consultations readily available, referral decisions could be made more easily and appropriately.

The committee recommends that physicians take more complete patient histories, particularly regarding personal and family histories, the onset of health problems, and occupational and environmental exposures. While there currently is grave concern about exposure to nerve agents during deployment in the Persian Gulf, other factors have an affect on psychological and neurological disorders. Patients can perform below expectations on neuropsychological tests for a number of reasons. In clinical assessments, therefore, it is important to rule out alternative causes of impairment. In addition, current and past exposures to occupational and environmental toxicants are important. Detailed histories are a valuable tool in identifying the etiology of a patient's problems.

The committee recommends that, to the extent possible, predeployment physical examinations given to members of the armed forces should be standardized among the services. The lack of uniform baseline information about service members makes diagnosis and treatment of postdeployment problems more difficult. To the extent that adequate baseline information is unavailable, physicians must rely on self-reporting. Adequate predeployment physical examinations, standardized across services, could prove an important tool for both clinical assessment and structured research.

The committee recommends that DoD increase the uniformity of CCEP forms and reporting procedures across sites. The CCEP system would benefit from increased consistency and the knowledge that each service is collecting and using the same information. Currently, each branch of service and each facility use different forms to complete examinations, tests, and referrals. Increasing the consistency of such forms and procedures would provide a more reliable picture of the care given to patients in the CCEP. As was stated in the

1996 report on the *Health Consequences of Service During the Persian Gulf War*, it is extremely important to create a uniform, continuous, and retrievable medical record. In addition, the 1996 report stated that the information should be collected according to standardized procedures and maintained in a computer-accessible format (IOM, 1996b). The committee concurs with those findings.

For each patient, the physician should provide written evidence that all organ systems were evaluated. The CCEP primary care physicians examine patients, and, if there are problems requiring additional expertise, the patients are referred to specialists. This is standard medical practice used across the United States. It would be appropriate, however, for the CCEP primary care physicians to document that their evaluations covered all organ systems. The committee is not recommending the use of new or sophisticated testing mechanisms. It is reinforcing the importance of the components of the basic medical examination. This increased documentation could be completed by noting the organ systems evaluated and whether each was normal or abnormal. For those listed as abnormal, additional information could be provided.

The committee strongly urges the DoD to offer group education and counseling to soldiers and their families concerned about exposure to toxic agents. Following the revelation by the DoD of possible exposure to nerve agents due to the destruction of the munitions dump at Khamisiyah, approximately 20,000 service personnel received a letter from the DoD stating that their units were in the vicinity during the demolition. Each recipient was encouraged to contact an 800 number if he or she was experiencing health problems believed to be a result of service in the Persian Gulf. Given this revelation, there may be a heightened sense of insecurity and concern among Persian Gulf veterans and their families about possible exposure to nerve agents. Risk communication is an important clinical activity. Family and group counseling can address heightened concerns about exposure as well as other issues. Such an approach provides an appropriate public health mechanism for imparting information and addressing concerns and should be made available to all Persian Gulf veterans.

Although it is beyond the scope of the charge to this committee to determine whether low-level exposure to nerve agents causes long-term health effects, the committee believes strongly that this is an important research area that ought to be pursued. Most of the literature regarding health effects of exposure to nerve agents (i.e., sarin and cyclosarin) addresses exposures high enough to cause clinically observable effects. These clinical effects are well documented and include miosis, blurred vision, nausea, vomiting, muscular twitching, weakness, convulsions, and death. Little known research has been conducted regarding the long-term health effects of low levels of exposure to these nerve agents. The application of findings from research on organophosphate pesticide exposure to the area of nerve agent exposure has limitations. However, even in such pesticide studies, long-term health effects have been documented only for acutely poisoned individuals—that is, persons with immediate clinical symptoms.

The committee emphasizes that the CCEP is *not* an appropriate vehicle for scientifically assessing questions about long-term health effects of low levels of exposure to nerve agents. *The CCEP is a clinical treatment program, not a research protocol.* It is important, therefore, not to attempt to use the findings of the CCEP to answer research questions. Those questions must be addressed through rigorous scientific research.

The committee notes that the CCEP could be useful in identifying promising directions for separate research studies. Examinations of the health effects—if any—of various wartime exposures have been hampered by poor information about the level of exposure and an inability to identify the individuals who may have been exposed. It is often difficult to retrospectively estimate exposure levels. However, information about where individuals were and when they were there could be combined with data regarding the presence of an exposure to develop surrogate measures. These surrogate measures could then be linked to health information and used to examine potential associations between exposures and health effects.

Although data from the CCEP cannot be used to *test* for associations, it can be combined with other information to help identify areas for future research. For example, the DoD identified approximately 20,000 service people belonging to units that were within a 50-kilometer radius of Khamisiyah at the time of the munitions demolition. Examining the health records of these people may yield insights into whether those who participated in the CCEP (or a similar program administered by the VA) have different illnesses or patterns of illnesses than do CCEP participants outside the 50-kilometer radius. More detailed discrimination of proximity to Khamisiyah (e.g., within 20 kilometers or within the units directly responsible for the munitions destruction) may provide additional information.

It is important, however, to understand the limitations of such comparisons. The results cannot be taken as research findings and generalized to the entire population of those deployed to the Persian Gulf. Active-duty military personnel participating in the DoD health registry may be either more or less healthy than other nonparticipants on active duty. CCEP comparisons on this self-selected group of patients should not be used to draw conclusions about the entire population of Persian Gulf veterans.

More broadly, the committee notes that information that helps to identify where individuals were in the Persian Gulf and when they were there will also facilitate research into potential service-related health problems. This information is currently needed to address the question of who might have been exposed to nerve agents and who could be part of the (unexposed) comparison groups necessary for epidemiological studies. Such information could also be used to more quickly and easily identify the exposed and unexposed groups that would be required to assess any future concerns regarding this or other exposures.

Generating geographical and temporal information for all 700,000 people who served in the Persian Gulf would be an immense endeavor. It would not be prudent to undertake such a task without first thoroughly understanding the effort required to complete it. It would, however, be appropriate to take steps now to identify and preserve records that could assist in the generation of such a database in the future. Records-based information is intrinsically superior to personal recollections, especially several years after the fact.

COMMITTEE ON THE EVALUATION OF THE DoD COMPREHENSIVE CLINICAL EVALUATION PROGRAM

Dan G. Blazer,* *Chair,* Dean of Medical Education and Professor of Psychiatry, Duke University Medical Center, Durham, North Carolina

Margit L. Bleecker, Director of the Center for Occupational and Environmental Neurology, Baltimore, Maryland

Evelyn J. Bromet, Professor, Department of Psychiatry, State University of New York at Stony Brook, Stony Brook, New York

Gerard Burrow,* Dean, Yale University School of Medicine, New Haven, Connecticut

Howard Kipen, Associate Professor and Director, Occupational Health Division, Robert Wood Johnson Medical School, Piscataway, New Jersey

Adel A. Mahmoud,* Chairman, Department of Medicine, Case Western Reserve University and University Hospitals of Cleveland, Cleveland, Ohio

Robert S. Pynoos, Associate Professor of Psychiatry and Dean of the Trauma Psychiatry Service, University of California at Los Angeles, Los Angeles, California

Guthrie L. Turner, Chief Medical Consultant, Office of Disability Determination Services, State of Washington, Tummwater, Washington

Michael Weisman, Professor, Division of Rheumatology, University of California at San Diego Medical Center, San Diego, California

Staff

Lyla M. Hernandez, Study Director

Sanjay S. Baliga, Research Associate

---

*Member, Institute of Medicine.

David A. Butler, Senior Program Officer
Donna M. Livingston, Project Assistant
James A. Bowers, Project Assistant
Kathleen R. Stratton, Director, Division of Health Promotion and Disease Prevention
Constance M. Pechura, Director, Division of Neuroscience and Behavioral Health

Appendix E

Adequacy of the Comprehensive Clinical Evaluation Program: A Focused Assessment*

CONCLUSIONS AND RECOMMENDATIONS

A great deal of time and effort has been expended evaluating DoD's Comprehensive Clinical Evaluation Program. It has been reviewed by the President's Advisory Committee, the General Accounting Office, the Office of Technology Assessment, the Institute of Medicine, and many other organizations. As more is learned, it becomes easier to focus on the kinds of questions the CCEP should be asking. As Dr. Penelope Keyl said in her workshop presentation on the development of good screening instruments, progress made over time will necessitate new generations of screening instruments. This does not imply that the first instrument developed is bad, but rather that time leads to new knowledge, which leads to the ability to improve the instrument.

Such is the case with the CCEP. Over time, the CCEP and other programs have generated information that has led us to focus on areas of importance for those concerned about the health consequences of Persian Gulf deployment. This information has enabled us to take a closer look, to make a more thorough examination of the system, and to identify areas in which change will be of benefit. The committee believes that such change is healthy, that it reflects growth, and that it should be a natural part of any system having as one of its goals the delivery of high-quality health care services.

---

*This appendix is excerpted from the Institute of Medicine report, *Adequacy of the Comprehensive Clinical Evaluation Program: A Focused Assessment*, Washington, D.C.: National Academy Press, 1997.

Change also occurs with individuals. It may be that as time passes or new information is released, some of those who have already participated in the CCEP will develop new concerns or problems. The committee hopes that DoD will encourage these individuals to return to the CCEP for further evaluation and diagnosis.

The committee wishes to emphasize that it is impressed with the dedication and concern exhibited by DoD personnel with whom committee members met. These individuals are knowledgeable regarding Persian Gulf issues and willing to learn more about identifying and resolving areas of concern for improving the health of active-duty personnel deployed to the Gulf.

MEDICALLY UNEXPLAINED SYMPTOM SYNDROMES

The committee spent some time deliberating on the precise meaning of "difficult to diagnose" or "ill defined" as a description of a category of conditions. When labeling something as difficult to diagnose, one usually means that special expertise is required to arrive at a diagnosis, but many of these conditions do not require such expertise. Chronic fatigue syndrome, fibromyalgia, and multiple chemical sensitivity are symptom complexes that have a great deal of overlap in the symptoms present in each condition but are well defined clinically, even if they are medically unexplained. Despite the fact that they are medically unexplained, they may cause significant impairment and they are illnesses that are only understood through time, that is, it requires the passage of time and the evaluation of responses to treatment to arrive at these diagnoses. The committee decided, therefore, to refer to this spectrum of illnesses as *medically unexplained symptom syndromes.* This spectrum of illnesses may include those which are etiologically unexplained, lack currently detectable pathophysiological changes, and/or cannot currently be diagnostically labeled.

These medically unexplained symptom syndromes are often associated with depression and anxiety. There remains a debate about how to distinguish these syndromes from psychiatric diagnoses, but it is clear that they are not simply psychiatric diagnoses. However, since most of the recommended treatments for medically unexplained symptom syndromes overlap with the pharmacological and behavioral treatments for psychological conditions or psychiatric diagnoses, the committee believes that it is important to identify and evaluate the symptoms associated with these conditions and then treat those symptoms.

The committee recommends that when patients presenting with medically unexplained symptom syndromes are evaluated, the provider must have access to the full and complete medical record, including previous use of services. The presence of such information is important because adequate evaluation of these disorders involves a longitudinal perspective that includes response to treatment.

In the area of medically unexplained symptom syndromes, it is sometimes not possible to arrive at a definitive diagnosis. It may be possible, however, to treat the presenting complaints or symptoms. **The committee recommends that in cases where a diagnosis cannot be identified, treatment should be targeted to specific symptoms or syndromes (e.g., fatigue, pain, depression).** If these symptoms and conditions are left untreated, they can become chronic and potentially disabling. **The committee recommends that the CCEP be encouraged to identify patients in this spectrum of illnesses early in the process of their disease. In addition, primary care providers should identify the patients' functional impairments so as to be able to suggest treatments that will help improve these disabilities.**

STRESS

In this group of medically unexplained symptom syndromes it is important to recognize and acknowledge that the problems and stress facing the patient will continue to be difficult. Stress is a major issue in the lives of patients within this spectrum of illness. Stress need not be looked at so much as a causative agent, but rather as a part of the condition of the patient that cannot be ignored. With these medically unexplained symptom syndromes, the potential for stress proliferation is great among both the person deployed to the Persian Gulf and the family members.

Media attention and reports by the military to Gulf War veterans that toxic exposure could have occurred are very stressful events, regardless of anyone's efforts to explain what happened. Such announcements carry with them stressful burdens for the veteran. The stress associated with these reports of and worry over toxic exposures needs to be recognized and addressed.

Research has shown that stressors have been associated with major depression, substance abuse, and various physical health problems. Those deployed to the Gulf were exposed to a vast array of different stressors that carry with them their own potential health consequences. Current collection of exposure information does not adequately address an investigation of traumatic events to which the deployed soldier may have been exposed. **The committee recommends that the CCEP contain questions on traumatic event exposures in addition to the exposure information currently being collected. This would include the addition of open-ended questions that ask the patient to list the events that were most upsetting to him or her while deployed. Positive responses to questions regarding such events, as well as to other exposure questions, should be pursued with a *narrative inquiry*, which would address such items as the specific nature of the exposure; the**

duration; the frequency of repetition; the dose or intensity (if appropriate); whether the patient was taking protective measures and, if so, what these measures were; and the symptoms manifested.

Other suggestions for questions that could be added to the CCEP include the following: When did you first have questions or worries about being exposed? When did you first hear other information on possible exposures? What were your responses to that information? Providers in the CCEP need to take a history that includes some narrative to allow the veteran to express how he or she feels.

It is always important to understand and acknowledge that the patients' complaints are real. It is certainly important for providers in the CCEP to do so when attempting to identify and address the health concerns of Persian Gulf veterans. Furthermore, no matter what additional information may be forthcoming about potential exposures to toxins and their effects, **the committee recommends that DoD providers acknowledge stressors as a legitimate but not necessarily sole cause of physical symptoms and conditions.**

The committee believes that there are certain jobs undertaken in the midst of war that, by their very nature, result in high stress (e.g., grave registration duty). The effect of stress associated with these jobs can be mitigated if approached properly. **The committee recommends that the DoD provide special training and debriefing for those who are engaged in high-risk jobs such as those associated with the Persian Gulf experience.** Every soldier who goes to war will be subjected to major disturbing events since war by its very nature involves death and destruction. **The committee recommends that DoD provide to each about-to-be deployed soldier risk or hazard communication which is well developed and designed to provide information regarding what the individual can expect and the potentially traumatic events to which he or she might be exposed.**

The committee wishes to emphasize that the accurate diagnosis of patients with medically unexplained symptom syndromes and/or conditions induced or exacerbated by upsetting events requires the expenditure of time, time in which the provider and the patient interact. It is not possible to hand the patient a questionnaire and expect that all necessary information will be revealed. In a world of time constraints and tightly scheduled appointments, **the committee recommends that adequate time must be provided during initial interactions with patients in the CCEP in order to ensure that all pertinent information is forthcoming.** The committee believes that the patient-physician interaction should be fostered, and the perception that evaluation is directed by the clock should be avoided.

SCREENING

Depression is a condition that is common in primary care. Most individuals who experience depression continue to function, but if they are left untreated, their conditio deteriorates. Unlike many of the medically unexplained symptom syı. ›mes, there are effective treatments for depression. The data presented indicate rising rates of depression among those examined in the CCEP but no evidence that individuals are being properly diagnosed or treated according to currently accepted clinical practice guidelines. There are many self-rated screening tests (e.g., the Beck Depression Inventory [BDI], the Zung Scale, the Center for Epidemiological Studies-Depression Scale [CES-D], the Inventory to Diagnose Depression [IDD]) that could be used as a first-level screen at the primary care level.

The committee recommends that there be increased screening at the primary care level for depression. Every primary care physician should have a simple standardized screen for depression. If a patient scores in the significant range, this person should be referred to a qualified mental health professional for further evaluation and treatment. If depression is identified, there has to be more questioning on exposure to traumatic problems.

There has been a great deal of concern evinced about the possibility of widespread PSTD in those deployed to the Persian Gulf. Most of the individuals identified as having PTSD are diagnosed following a structured interview at Phase II. However, the committee believes that there are those who have *some* of the symptoms of PTSD or of depression but are not true PTSD cases yet might be helped with treatment of their symptoms.

The committee recommends that any individual who reports any significant PTSD symptoms and/or a significant traumatic stressor should be referred to a qualified mental health professional for further evaluation and treatment.

Substance abuse or misuse problems are prevalent in primary care. In addition, individuals with untreated depression or with medically unexplained symptom syndromes may have an enhanced risk of substance abuse. (See Appendix I for examples of screening instruments.) **The committee recommends, therefore, that every primary care physician should have a simple, standardized screen for substance abuse. Every individual who screens positive should be referred for further treatment and evaluation.**

There are certain areas in which baseline assessments are of immense value in the clinical evaluation of an individual patient's status (e.g., pulmonary function and neurobehavioral testing). Changes in neurocognitive and peripheral nerve function are measured by comparing the individual's current status to a baseline measure. This is also true for measuring complaints of memory impairment. Individual baseline information is necessary because the variability across individuals is too great to identify a generalized "normal" screening level.

The committee recommends that DoD explore the possibility of using neurobehavioral testing at entry into the military to determine whether it is feasible to use such tests to predict change in functioning or track change in function during a soldier's military career.

PROGRAM EVALUATION

Most patients in the CCEP receive a diagnosis after completing a Phase I examination; some are referred to Phase II for evaluation; and a few have gone on to participate in the program at the Specialized Care Center. Information presented to the committee indicates that there is great variation across regions in the percentage of patients who are diagnosed as having primary psychiatric diagnoses. A determination of the reasons for this variation should be made. Although there may be many reasons, one explanation could relate to the consistency with which procedures for diagnosis and referral are implemented from facility to facility. **The committee recommends that an evaluation be conducted to examine (1) the consistency with which Phase I examinations are conducted across facilities; (2) the patterns of referral from Phase I to Phase II; and (3) the adequacy of treatment provided to certain categories of patients where there is the potential for great impact on patient outcomes when effective treatment is rendered (e.g., depression).**

This effort could be facilitated by the development and use of clinical practice guidelines such as those currently being developed by the Department of Veterans Affairs and many medical specialties. Clinical practice guidelines are systematically developed statements that assist practitioners and patients in decision making about appropriate health care for specific clinical circumstances (IOM, 1992). The process of developing these guidelines could also serve as an opportunity for increased learning for providers since their participation is crucial to successful implementation.

The Specialized Care Center at Walter Reed Army Medical Center has provided evaluation and treatment to 78 patients. A great deal of effort and thought has gone into the development of a program designed to help the patient understand his or her conditions and engage in behaviors most likely to result in improvement. The committee was asked to assess the effectiveness of this center within the context of medically unexplained symptom syndromes, stress, and psychiatric disorders. As the committee began its discussion of the effectiveness of the Specialized Care Center it became apparent that such an assessment was dependent on a number of factors that have not been well defined. What is the goal of the center—is it treatment, research, or education? Should a major consideration in the center's evaluation be the cost of services?

Should the numbers of those receiving care be taken into consideration, and if so, what are the barriers to patients accessing this level of care?

The committee concluded that at this time, it is not possible to conduct a fair or adequate evaluation of the Specialized Care Center. **The committee recommends that a short-term plan (perhaps 5 years) be developed for the Specialized Care Center that would specify goals and expected outcomes.** Based on such a plan, an evaluation could then be undertaken to assess the effectiveness of the center.

COORDINATION WITH THE VA

Given that many now receiving services in the DoD health care system will eventually move to the VA health care system, it is important to have good communication between DoD and the VA. This may be particularly true in the areas of medically unexplained symptom syndromes and psychiatric disorders, where accurate diagnosis and assessment of response to treatment are important for positive patient outcomes. **The committee recommends that DoD explore ways to increase communication with the VA, particularly as it relates to the ongoing treatment of patients.**

Both patients and providers would benefit from increased educational activity regarding Persian Gulf health issues. Provider turnover within DoD is a factor that must be taken into consideration when examining the special health needs and concerns of active-duty personnel who were deployed to the Persian Gulf. Although efforts at provider education were extensive at the time the CCEP was implemented, three years have passed and many new providers have entered the system. These individuals should be oriented to the special needs, concerns, and procedures involved, and all providers should be updated regularly.

The VA has developed a number of approaches to provider education. Interactive satellite teleconferences are available periodically for medical center staff to discuss particular issues of concern. The VA conducts quarterly national telephone conference calls, directs periodic educational mailings to Persian Gulf Registry providers in each health facility, and conducts an annual conference on the health consequences of Persian Gulf service. **The committee recommends that DoD examine the activities and materials for provider education developed by the VA to determine if some of the items might be used as educational approaches for DoD providers.**

Although the topics of ongoing educational efforts are best determined by DoD on a periodic basis, **the committee recommends that DoD mount an effort designed to educate providers to the fact that conditions related to stress are not necessarily psychiatric conditions. The committee recommends that depression be a topic of education for all primary care**

providers, with emphasis on the facts that depression is common, it is treatable, and individuals who experience depression can continue to function.

The committee wishes to reemphasize the fact that the CCEP is not a research protocol but rather a program designed to diagnose the health problems of those who served in the Persian Gulf. As such, information obtained through the CCEP should not be used to answer research questions. It is appropriate, however, to use the data and narrative information obtained from the CCEP to inform the clinical treatment process. In doing so, the committee believes that it is important to unbundle diagnostic categories. For example, tension headache is classified as a somatoform disorder within the category of psychiatric diagnosis.

In addition, a tremendous amount of qualitative information could be used in developing case studies to help providers better understand diagnostic and treatment approaches that appear effective at improving individual patients' conditions.

The committee recommends that CCEP information be used to develop case studies that will help educate providers about Persian Gulf health problems. There are a number of ways in which these case studies could be shared including presentation during professional meetings.

There is also a need for education and communication with individuals who were deployed to the Gulf and with their families. These individuals are concerned about the potential impact of Persian Gulf deployment on their health, whether or not their health concerns will affect their military careers, their ability to obtain health insurance once they leave the service, and a number of other issues that need to be addressed.

A variety of mechanisms are available for providing such information including individual post newsletters, the Internet, mailings to those in the Registry, and public forums. It is especially important to provide a forum for discussion each time new information is released on possible exposures. **The committee recommends that DoD develop approaches to communication and education that address the concerns of individuals deployed to the Persian Gulf and their families.**

Appendix F

VA Phase I Protocol

PROTOCOL FOR CONDUCTING THE PHYSICAL EXAMINATION AND ORDERING DIAGNOSTIC STUDIES

1. It is essential that a complete medical history, physical examination and interview be performed and documented on appropriate forms. The required forms that must be fully completed are: Standard Form (SF) 88, Report of Medical Examination, Department of Veterans Affairs (VA) Form 10-9009A, Persian Gulf Registry Code Sheet, and SF 509, Progress Notes (for follow-up). These are to be maintained in the veteran's Consolidated Health Record (CHR). NOTE: *This should be accomplished by or under the direct supervision of the Veterans' Registry Physician (VRP). Examination data will be recorded in the veteran's medical record as routinely as done for any other medical examination.* The complete medical history should address the following:

(a) Family history;
(b) Occupational history;
(c) Social history including tobacco, alcohol, drug use;
(d) Civilian exposure(s) history to possible toxic agents;
(e) Psychosocial history; and
(f) Review of systems.

2. The person actually performing the physical examination will be identified by name, signature and title (i.e., Doctor of Osteopathy, Doctor of Medicine, Physician's Assistant, etc.). A physician's countersignature is

required if the examiner is other than a physician. Under normal circumstances, VRP will provide such countersignatures.

3. When a Persian Gulf Registry (PGR) examination is done as part of a compensation and pension examination, the physical examination will be done by/or under the direct supervision of the VRP.

4. The physician should be aware of the variety of exposures endemic to the Persian Gulf area. These are listed in Appendix 2C and on VA Form 10-90009A. There has been a wide distribution of major categories of diagnosis reported by VA VRPs; however, no significant variation in occurrence of major categories of medical problems has been identified. We are listing below (for informational purposes) some of the health problems and/or disease which should be considered:

NOTE: Unfortunately the International Classification of Diseases, 9th Edition, Clinical Modification (ICD-9-CM) coding systems does not give sufficient codes to correctly identify all symptoms and diagnoses. A number of diagnoses that have been reported by Veterans' Registry Physicians do not have ICD-9-CM codes for specific identification in the Veterans Health Administration (VHA)s database. To correct this, three new codes have been created. They are Apnea, Sleep (99001), Chronic Fatigue Syndrome (CFS) (99002), and Fibromyalgia (99003). Make certain these codes are used when completing the Persian Gulf Registry code sheets for patients who have these diagnoses. As a result of inadequate coding designations, there has been confusion between the symptoms (complaints) and diagnoses listed on the PGR code sheets. Example one: Arthralgia (diagnostic code 7194) has been used for the symptom "pain in the joint," where the symptom code 7819 (other symptoms involving nervous and musculoskeletal systems) would be more appropriate. Example two: Symptom ICD-9-CM code 78051 has been designated for insomnia with sleep apnea; however, sleep apnea is more correctly identified as a specific diagnosis which has the new code 99001. Symptom code 78051 may still be used for insomnia with sleep apnea. Example three: Symptom ICD-9-CM code 7807 has been used to designate CFS and the symptoms of malaise and fatigue. The new code 99002 has been determined for CFS, so ICD-9-CM code 7807 should be used for medical complaints of malaise and fatigue.

Diagnoses		International Classification of Diseases ICD-9-CM Codes
(1)	Amebiasis	006
(2)	Apnea, sleep	99001
(3)	Arthralgia	7194
(4)	Asthma	493
(5)	Brill's Zinsser disease (recrudescent typhus)	0811
(6)	Bronchiectasis	494
(7)	Bronchopneumonia, organism unspecified	485
(8)	Brucellosis	023
(9)	Chronic obstructive pulmonary disease, not elsewhere classified	496
(10)	Chronic bronchitis	491
(11)	Chronic Fatigue Syndrome	99002
(12)	Chronic Laryngotracheitis	4761
(13)	Chronic respiratory conditions due to fumes and vapors	5064
(14)	Emphysema	492
(15)	Fibromyalgia	99003
(16)	Giardiasis	0071
(17)	Leishmaniasis	085
(18)	Malaria	084
(19)	Other and unspecified diseases of upper respiratory tract	4789
(20)	Pneumoconiosis due to other silica or silicates	502
(21)	Pneumoconiosis, unspecified	505
(22)	Unspecified chronic respiratory disease	5199
(23)	Respiratory conditions due to unspecified external agent	5089
(24)	Sandfly fever (phlebatomus fever)	0660
(25)	Schistosomiasis (bilharziasis)	120
(26)	Toxoplasmosis	130
(27)	Typhoid fever, also carrier—V02.1	0020
(28)	Tuberculosis, specify variant(s)	010–018
(29)	Viral hepatitis	070
(30)	Memory loss	310
(31)	Polyneuropathy	356–357
(32)	Skin rash	680–709
(33)	Adjustment disorder, including Post Traumatic Stress Disorder (PTSD)	309
(34)	Alcohol dependence syndrome	303
(35)	Drug dependence	304

5. In gathering these data, it is important to determine and record, the:
   a. Time of onset of the symptoms or conditions,
   b. Intensity,
   c. Degree of physical incapacitation, and
   d. Details of any treatment received.

6. Each veteran will be given the following baseline laboratory studies (Phase I Registry Examination):
   a. Complete Blood Count (CBC);
   b. Electrolyte Glucose (SMA-6, SMA-12), or equivalent blood chemistries and enzyme studies; and
   c. Urinalysis.

7. Appropriate additional diagnostic studies should be performed and consultations obtained as indicated by the patient's symptoms and the physical and laboratory findings. *NOTE: If individuals have unexplained illnesses, after a Phase I registry examination is performed, a Phase II examination is mandated (See Ch. 3, App 3A, for instructions.)*
   a. Other diagnostic studies, such as pulmonary function tests, sperm counts, should be performed if medically indicated.
   b. Laboratory tests results should be filed in the CHR.

Appendix G

VA Phase II Protocol

UNIFORM CASE ASSESSMENT PROTOCOL (UCAP)

1. Phase I Level Laboratory Evaluations
   a. Complete Blood Count (CBC)
   b. Urinalysis, and
   c. Blood Chemistry—SMA-6

2. Phase II—Level Evaluation Protocol. Phase II Level Evaluations are recommended for those veterans after complete clinically indicated evaluations are conducted and the physician determines that the patient has an unexplained illness. Individuals who after completing Phase I or Registry evaluations, have a disability and do not have a clearly defined diagnosis which explains their symptoms, must receive the following supplemental baseline laboratory tests and consultations.

   a. Supplemental Baseline Laboratory Tests
      (1) CBC,
      (2) Sedimentation Rate Erythrocyte Sedimentation Rate (ESR),
      (3) C-Reactive Protein,
      (4) Rheumatoid Factor,
      (5) Anti-Nuclear Antibody (ANA),
      (6) Liver Function,
      (7) Creatine Phosphokinase (CPK),
      (8) Hepatitis Serology,

(9) Human Immunodeficiency (HIV),
(10) Venereal Disease Research Laboratory (VDRL),
(11) B-12 and Folate,
(12) Thyroid Function Test,
(13) Urinalysis, and
(14) Tuberculosis (TB) Skin Test Purified Protein Derivative (PPD).

b. Consultations to include:
(1) Dental, but only if participant's annual screening is not done.
(2) Infectious Disease.
(3) Psychiatry, but only with physician administered instrument.
(a) Structured Clinical Interview for the *Diagnostic and Statistical Manual of Mental Disorders*, Third Edition Revised (DSM III-R). **NOTE**: *Delete modules for mania and psychosis.*
(b) Clinician Administered Post Traumatic Stress Disorder (PTSD) Scale (CAPS).
(4) Neuropsychological Testing, but only as indicated by a psychiatry consult.

c. Symptom-Specific Examination. Individuals who have the following symptoms should have the listed minimum work-up.
(1) Diarrhea, to include:
(a) Gastrointestinal (GI) consults,
(b) Stool for Ova and Parasites (O&P),
(c) Stool Leukocytes,
(d) Stool Culture,
(e) Stool Volume,
(f) Colonoscopy with biopsies, and
(g) Esophagastroduodenoscopy (EGD) with biopsies and aspiration.
(2) Abdominal pain to include:
(a) GI consult,
(b) EGD with biopsy and aspiration,
(c) Colonoscopy with biopsy,
(d) Abdominal ultrasound,
(e) Upper Gastrointestinal (UGI) series with small bowel follow-through, and
(f) Abdominal Computed Tomography (CT) Scan.
(3) Headache
(a) Magnetic Resonance Imaging (MRI) of the head, and
(b) Lumbar Puncture (LP) to include:
1. Glucose,
2. Protein,

3. Cell Count,
4. VDRL,
5. Oligoclonal (lgG),
6. Myelin basic protein,
7. Opening pressure, and
8. Neurology

(4) Muscle Aches and/or Numbness
(a) Electromyogram (EMG), and
(b) Nerve Conduction Velocity (NCV).

(5) Memory Loss, only if verified by neuropsychological testing, to include:
(a) Magnetic Resonance Imaging (MRI),
(b) LP, **NOTE**: *See tests on headache evaluation.*
(c) Neurology consult,
(d) Neuro-psychological testing.

(6) Vertigo and/or Tinnitus, to include:
(a) Audiogram,
(b) Electronystamogram (ENG), and
(c) Brainstem Auditory Evoked Response (BAER).

(7) Chronic Fatigue, to include:
(a) Polysomnography, and
(b) Multiple Sleep Latency Test (MSLT).

(8) Chronic Cough and/or Shortness of Breath, to include:
(a) Pulmonary Consult,
(b) Pulmonary Function Test (PFT) with exercise and Arterial Blood Gases (ABG),
(c) If routine PFTs are negative, perform Methacholine challenge test, and
(d) Bronchoscopy with biopsy and/or lavage which is to be considered if PFTs are normal.

(9) Chest Pain and/or Palpitations, to include:
(a) Electrocardiogram (ECG),
(b) Exercise Stress Test, and
(c) Holter monitor.

(10) Skin Rash, to include:
(a) Dermatology consults, and
(b) Consider a biopsy.

(11) Reproductive Concerns, to include for:
(a) Males, an urology consult; and
(b) Females, a gynecology (GYN) consult.
(c) Additional elements recommended for the evaluation of Persian Gulf veterans with complaints of Reproductive Health Problems (RHP):

1. Detailed genitourinary history and/or problems, e.g.:
   a. Sexual,
   b. Genitourinary symptoms,
   c. Menstrual,
   d. Contraceptive practices,
   e. Pregnancy-related,
   f. Conception,
   g. Birth defects,
   h. Congenital disorders,
   i. Menopause,
   j. Prior infections,
   k. Prior surgery, and
   l. Exposures to toxic agents, etc.
2. Detailed genital/pelvic examination
3. Laboratory and ancillary testing, e.g.:
   a. Pap tests; and
   b. Tests for genitourinary infections.
4. Urologist consultations for male veterans who have RHP that cannot be diagnosed or managed successfully by primary care practitioners.
5. Gynecology consultation for female veterans who have RHP that cannot be diagnosed or managed successfully by primary care practitioners.

(d) Additional elements for evaluation of Persian Gulf veterans with complaints of infertility.

1. Detailed menstrual and reproductive history (such as the infertility questionnaire utilized by Walter Reed Army Medical Center*).
2. Semen analysis, e.g.:
   a. Volume,
   b. pH,
   c. Liquefaction,
   d. Sperm concentration,
   e. Motility,
   f. Progressive motility,
   g. Sperm viability,
   h. Leukocytes, and
   i. Morphology.
3. Referral to an infertility specialist or program.

(e) Additional elements for evaluation of Persian Gulf veterans with complaints related to birth defects or genetic disorders in offspring conceived during or after Persian Gulf service.

1. Detailed history of congenital or genetic disorders (such as the Patient Genetic Screen Questionnaire utilized by Walter Reed Army Medical Center*).
2. Detailed occupational exposures questionnaire (such as Worker and Supervisor Questionnaires utilized by National Naval Medical Center*).
3. Referral to a genetic disease specialist or program.

**For copies of these questionnaires (Items d-1 and e-1 and 2), contact VA Environmental Agents Service (103A) at 202-565-4183.*

Appendix H

Persian Gulf Registry Code Sheet

Department of Veterans Affairs

PERSIAN GULF REGISTRY CODE SHEET

TT # 1 | 1. Use PTF Number Only | FACILITY NO. (2) (3) (4) | SUFFIX (5) (6) (7)

PART 1 (Phase I)

The information the veteran supplies may be disclosed outside the VA to Federal, State and local government agencies and National Health Organizations to assist in the development of programs for research purposes and other uses as stated in the "Notice of Systems of VA Records" published in the Federal Register in accordance with the Privacy Act of 1974

INSTRUCTIONS: Please print. Use only one letter or number per block. If possible use black ballpoint or felt-tip pen. Shaded areas for VA use only. (DO NOT USE BLUE INK)

2. LAST NAME (8-33)

3. FIRST NAME (34-48) | 4. MIDDLE NAME (49-58) | 5. TYPE (59)

6. SOCIAL SECURITY NUMBER (60-69) (60) | 7. D.O.B. (Complete all blanks) MO (70-71) DAY (72-73) YR (74-75)

8. ADDRESS (Street Name and Apartment Number, if applicable) 76-101

8A. CITY OR TOWN (102-127)

8B. COUNTY | STATE | 8C. ZIP CODE (128-132) | 8D. LEAVE BLANK (133) (134) (135) (136) | 8E. COUNTY (137-139) | STATE (140-141)

9. RACE/ETHNICITY (Enter one code at right) 142
1=American Indian or Alaskan Native 3=Black, Not of Hispanic Origin 5=Hispanic
2=Asian or Pacific Islander 4=White, Not of Hispanic Origin 6=Unknown

10. MARITAL STATUS (Enter one code at right) 143
1=Married 3=Separated 5=Single, Never Married
2=Divorced 4=Widowed

11. SEX (Enter one code at right) M=Male F=Female 144

12. CURRENT STATUS (Enter one code at right) 145
1 = Inpatient 3 = Incarcerated 5=Active Duty (Inpatient)
2 = Outpatient 4 = Active Duty (Outpatient)

13. BRANCH OF SERVICE (If more than one, enter latest Persian Gulf Service) 146
1=Army 3=Navy 5=Coast Guard
2=Air Force 4=Marine Corps 6=Other

14. DID VETERAN HAVE MILITARY SERVICE IN PERSIAN GULF AREA? 147
Y=Yes (If "Yes", list below the dates of veteran's last two periods of service there) N=No (If "No", Persian Gulf Veterans not eligible for PGR exam.

A. LAST PERIOD | FROM MO (148-149) YR (150-151) | TO MO (152-153) YR (154-155) | B. NEXT TO LAST PERIOD | FROM MO (156-157) YR (158-159) | TO MO (160-161) YR (162-163)

15A. IN WHAT AREAS DID VETERAN SERVE? (Enter appropriate code in block 164) 164
1 = Combat Zone
2 = Other Land Area
3 = Sea Duty

15B. IF OTHER SERVICE OR "DON'T KNOW" (Enter appropriate code in block 164) 165
4 = Other (Specify i.e. Air Force, Ground or Air Crew, etc.)
5 = Don't Know

16. MILITARY UNITS AND MOS

16A. LIST MILITARY UNITS IN WHICH VETERAN SERVED. PLEASE SPECIFY COMPLETE UNABBREVIATED TITLE. (Company, battalion, etc.)

16B. LIST MILITARY OCCUPATIONAL SPECIALTY (MOS)

16C. WERE ACTUAL DUTIES DIFFERENT FROM MOS? ENTER EITHER OF THE FOLLOWING CODES IN BLOCK 166 166
Y = Yes N = No

16D. IF YES, LIST HERE AND IN CONSOLIDATED HEALTH RECORD

16E. ENTER THE NAME OF THE UNIT IN WHICH VETERAN HAD THE LONGEST AND NEXT TO LONGEST PERIOD OF SERVICE WHILE IN THE PERSIAN GULF

NOTE A&E: These units could be different from the one to which the veterans was assigned if veterans was on detached duty.

17. ENTER THE DATES OF THE LAST TWO PERIODS OF SERVICE (If different from above)

A. LAST PERIOD | FROM MO (167-168) YR (169-170) | TO MO (171-172) YR (173-174) | B. NEXT TO LAST PERIOD | FROM MO (175-176) YR (177-178) | TO MO (179-180) YR (181-182)

VA FORM JUL 1995 10–9009a(RS)

NAME: ____________________

SSN: ____________________

18.	VETERANS EXPOSURE TO ENVIRONMENTAL FACTORS (ENTER APPROPRIATE CODES)		
18A.	ARE YOU CURRENTLY SMOKING CIGARETTES? ENTER ONE OF THE FOLLOWING CODES IN BLOCK 183. IF NO, GO TO ITEM 18D.	Y=YES N=NO	(183)
18B.	IF YES, HOW MANY YEARS HAVE YOU BEEN SMOKING CIGARETTES? ENTER THE NUMBER OF YEARS IN BLOCK 184 AND 185.		(184) (185)
18C.	ON THE AVERAGE HOW MANY PACKS ARE YOU SMOKING PER DAY? ENTER THE NUMBER OF PACKS IN BLOCKS 186 AND 187		(186) (187)
18D.	HAVE YOU SMOKED CIGARETTES IN THE PAST? ENTER ONE OF THE FOLLOWING CODES IN BLOCK 188. IF NO, GO TO ITEM 18G.	Y=YES N=NO	(188)
18E.	IF YES, HOW MANY YEARS HAD YOU SMOKED? ENTER NUMBER OF YEARS IN BLOCKS 189 AND 190.		(189) (190)
18F.	ON THE AVERAGE, HOW MANY PACKS DID YOU SMOKE PER DAY? ENTER THE NUMBER OF PACKS IN BLOCKS 191 AND 192.		(191) (192)
18G-Z1.	WHILE IN THE PERSIAN GULF DO YOU BELIEVE YOU WERE EXPOSED TO ANY OF THE FOLLOWING:		
18G.	SMOKE FROM OIL FIRES? ENTER ONE OF THE FOLLOWING CODES IN BLOCK 193.	Y=YES N=NO U=UNKNOWN	(193)
18H.	SMOKE OR FUMES FROM TENT HEATERS? ENTER ONE OF THE FOLLOWING CODES IN BLOCK 194.	Y=YES N=NO U=UNKNOWN	(194)
18I.	CIGARETTE SMOKE (PASSIVE) FROM OTHERS? ENTER ONE OF THE FOLLOWING CODES IN BLOCK 195.	Y=YES N=NO U=UNKNOWN	(195)
18J.	DIESEL AND/OR OTHER PETROCHEMICAL FUMES? ENTER ONE OF THE FOLLOWING CODES IN BLOCK 196.	Y=YES N=NO U=UNKNOWN	(196)
18K.	EXPOSURE TO BURNING TRASH/FECES? ENTER ONE OF THE FOLLOWING CODES IN BLOCK 197.	Y=YES N=NO U=UNKNOWN	(197)
18L.	SKIN EXPOSURE TO DIESEL OR OTHER PETROCHEMICAL FUEL? ENTER ONE OF THE FOLLOWING CODES IN BLOCK 198.	Y=YES N=NO U=UNKNOWN	(198)
18M.	CARC (CHEMICAL AGENT RESISTANT COMPOUND)? ENTER ONE OF THE FOLLOWING CODES IN BLOCK 199.	Y=YES N=NO U=UNKNOWN	(199)
18N.	OTHER PAINTS AND/OR SOLVENTS AND/OR PETROCHEMICAL SUBSTANCES? ENTER ONE OF THE FOLLOWING CODES IN BLOCK 200.	Y=YES N=NO U=UNKNOWN	(200)
18O.	DEPLETED URANIUM? ENTER ONE OF THE FOLLOWING CODES IN BLOCK 201.	Y=YES N=NO U=UNKNOWN	(201)
18P.	MICROWAVES? ENTER ONE OF THE FOLLOWING CODES IN BLOCK 202.	Y=YES N=NO U=UNKNOWN	(202)
18Q.	PERSONAL PESTICIDE USE, INCLUDING CREAMS, SPRAYS OR FLEA COLLARS? ENTER ONE OF THE FOLLOWING CODES IN BLOCK 203.	Y=YES N=NO U=UNKNOWN	(203)
18R.	NERVE GAS OR OTHER NERVE AGENTS? ENTER ONE OF THE FOLLOWING CODES IN BLOCK 204.	Y=YES N=NO U=UNKNOWN	(204)
18S.	DRUG (PYRIDOSTIGMINE) USED TO PROTECT AGAINST NERVE AGENTS? ENTER ONE OF THE FOLLOWING CODES IN BLOCK 205.	Y=YES N=NO U=UNKNOWN	(205)
18T.	MUSTARD GAS OR OTHER AGENTS? ENTER ONE OF THE FOLLOWING CODES IN BLOCK 206.	Y=YES N=NO U=UNKNOWN	(206)
18U.	ATE OR DRANK FOOD CONTAMINATED WITH SMOKE, OIL OR OTHER CHEMICAL? ENTER ONE OF THE FOLLOWING CODES IN BLOCK 207.	Y=YES N=NO U=UNKNOWN	(207)

NAME: ______________________

SSN: ______________________

18V. ATE FOOD OTHER THAN PROVIDE BY ARMED FORCES? ENTER ONE OF THE FOLLOWING CODES IN BLOCK 208.	Y=YES N=NO U=UNKNOWN	(208)
18W. BATHED IN OR DRANK WATER CONTAMINATED WITH SMOKE OR OTHER CHEMICAL? ENTER ONE OF THE FOLLOWING CODES IN BLOCK 209.	Y=YES N=NO U=UNKNOWN	(209)
18X. BATHED IN WATER OTHER THAN PROVIDED BY ARMED FORCES? ENTER ONE OF THE FOLLOWING CODES IN BLOCK 210.	Y=YES N=NO U=UNKNOWN	(210)
18Y. IMMUNIZATION AGAINST ANTHRAX? ENTER ONE OF THE FOLLOWING CODES IN BLOCK 211.	Y=YES N=NO U=UNKNOWN	(211)
18Z. IMMUNIZATION AGAINST BOTULISM? ENTER ONE OF THE FOLLOWING CODES IN BLOCK 212.	Y=YES N=NO U=UNKNOWN	(212)

18Z1. OTHER EXPOSURES? ENTER HERE AND IN CHR ONLY.

____

____

____

____

19. DID VETERAN HAVE ANY OF THE FOLLOWING EXPERIENCES WHILE IN THE PERSIAN GULF? ENTER APPROPRIATE CODE.		
19A. DID YOU EVER GO ON COMBAT PATROLS OR HAVE OTHER VERY DANGEROUS DUTY? ENTER ONE OF THE FOLLOWING CODES IN BLOCK 213. 1=NO 2=1-3X 3=4-12X 4=13-50X 5=51+ TIMES		(213)
19B. WERE YOU EVER UNDER ENEMY FIRE (INCLUDING "SCUDS")? ENTER ONE OF THE FOLLOWING CODES IN BLOCK 214. 1 = NEVER 2 = 1DAY 3 =< 1 WEEK 4 = 1-< 4WEEKS 5 = 4 WEEKS OR MORE		(214)
19C. WHAT PERCENTAGE OF PEOPLE IN YOUR UNIT WERE KILLED (KIA), WOUNDED OR MISSING IN ACTION (MIA), ENTER ONE OF THE FOLLOWING CODES IN BLOCK 215. 1=NONE 2=1-25% 3=26-50% 4=51-75% 5=76% OR MORE		(215)
19D. HOW OFTEN DID YOU SEE SOMEONE HIT BY INCOMING OR OUTGOING ROUNDS? ENTER ONE OF THE FOLLOWING CODES IN BLOCK 216. 1=NEVER 2=1-2X 3=3-12X 4=13-50X 5=51 OR MORE TIMES		(216)
19E. HOW OFTEN WERE YOU IN DANGER OF BEING INJURED OR KILLED (I.E. PINNED DOWN, OVERRUN, AMBUSHED, NEAR MISS, ETC.)? ENTER ONE OF THE FOLLOWING CODES IN BLOCK 217. 1=NEVER 2=1-2X 3=3-12X 4=13-50X 5=51 OR MORE TIMES		(217)
19F. DID YOU WITNESS CHEMICAL ALARMS? ENTER ONE OF THE FOLLOWING CODES IN BLOCK 218.	Y=YES N=NO U=UNKNOWN	(218)
20. VETERAN'S HEALTH (VETERAN'S EVALUATION)		
20A. WHICH BEST DESCRIBES VETERAN'S HEALTH AFTER PERSION GULF SERVICE? ENTER ONE OF THE FOLLOWING CODES IN BLOCK 219. 1 = Very Good 2 = Good 3 = Fair 4 = Poor 5 = Very Poor		(219)
21. VETERAN'S FUNCTIONAL IMPAIRMENT		
21A. WHICH BEST DESCRIBES VETERAN'S OWN ASSESSMENT OF FUNCTIONAL IMPAIRMENT? ENTER' ONE OF THE FOLLOWING CODES IN BLOCK 220. 1=NO IMPAIRMENT 2=SLIGHT IMPAIRMENT 3=MODERATE IMPAIRMENT 4=SEVERE IMPAIRMENT		(220)
21B. HOW MANY WORKDAYS WERE LOST BY VETERAN DUE TO ILLNESS IN THE PAST 90 DAYS? ENTER NUMBER OF DAYS LOST IN BLOCKS 221-222.	(221)	(222)
22. EVIDENCE OF BIRTH DEFECTS AND INFANT DEATH(S) AMONG VETERAN'S CHILDREN AND PROBLEMS WITH PREGNANCY AND INFERTILITY.		
22A. HOW MANY CHILDREN DOES VETERAN HAVE? ENTER NUMBER IN BLOCKS 223 AND 224. (I.E. 05). IF NONE, LEAVE BLANK AND GO TO ITEM 22C.	(223)	(224)

NAME: ____________________

SSN: ____________________

22B. HOW MANY OF THESE CHILDREN WERE BORN WITH BIRTH DEFECTS? (BIRTH DEFECTS ARE ANY STRUCTURAL, FUNCTIONAL, OR BIOCHEMICAL ABNORMALITY AT BIRTH WHETHER GENETICALLY DETERMINED OR INDUCED DURING GESTATION THAT IS NOT DUE TO INJURIES SUFFERED DURING BIRTH.) ENTER NUMBER IN BLOCKS 225 AND 226. IF NONE, GO TO ITEM 22C.		(225) (226)
22B1. HOW MANY OF THESE CHILDREN WERE CONCEIVED BEFORE GULF SERVICE? ENTER THE NUMBER OF CHILDREN IN BLOCKS 227 AND 228. IF NONE, LEAVE BLANK AND GO TO ITEM 22B2.		(227) (228)
22B1(a) STATE MATERNAL AGE AT CONCEPTION OF FIRST CHILD CONCEIVED BEFORE GULF SERVICE? ENTER AGE IN BLOCKS 229 AND 230.		(229) (230)
22B2. HOW MANY OF THESE CHILDREN WERE CONCEIVED DURING AND AFTER GULF SERVICE? ENTER NUMBER IN BLOCK 231 AND 232. IF NONE, LEAVE BLANK AND GO TO ITEM 22C.		(231) (232)
22B2(a) STATE MATERNAL AGE AT CONCEPTION OF FIRST CHILD CONCEIVED DURING AND AFTER GULF SERVICE? ENTER AGE IN BLOCKS 229 AND 230.		(233) (234)
22C. HAS VETERAN OR SPOUSE HAD INFERTILITY PROBLEMS? (INFERTILITY PROBLEMS OF VETERAN OR SPOUSE BECOMING PREGNANT. NOTE: INFERTILITY - RELATIVE STERILITY DEFINED AS INABILITY TO CONCEIVE AFTER 12 OR MORE MONTHS OF INTERCOURSE WITHOUT USE OF CONTRACEPTION AND WHEN NEITHER SPOUSE IS SURGICALLY STERILIZED.) ENTER ONE OF THE FOLLOWING CODES IN BLOCK 235. IF NO, GO TO ITEM 22D.	Y=YES N=NO	(235)
22C1. HAS VETERAN OR SPOUSE HAD INFERTILITY BEFORE GULF SERVICE? ENTER ONE OF THE FOLLOWING CODES IN BLOCK 236. IF NO, GO TO ITEM 22C2.	Y=YES N=NO	(236)
22C1(a). STATE MATERNAL AGE DURING FIRST ATTEMPTS TO CONCEIVE. ENTER AGE IN BLOCKS 237 AND 238.		(237) (238)
22C2. HAS VETERAN OR SPOUSE HAD INFERTILITY AFTER RETURN FROM GULF SERVICE? ENTER ONE OF THE FOLLOWING CODES IN BLOCK 239. IF NO, GO TO ITEM 22D.	Y=YES N=NO	(239)
22C2(a). STATE MATERNAL AGE DURING FIRST ATTEMPTS TO CONCEIVE. ENTER AGE IN BLOCKS 240 AND 241.		(240) (241)
22D. HAS VETERAN OR SPOUSE HAD MISCARRIAGE(S) (NOTE: MISCARRIAGES ARE SPONTANEOUS EXPLUSION OF THE PRODUCTS OF CONCEPTION BEFORE 20 WEEKS OF GESTATION - SPONTANEOUS ABORTION) ENTER ONE OF THE FOLLOWING CODES IN BLOCK 242. IF NO, GO TO ITEM 22E.	Y=YES N=NO	(242)
22D1. HAS VETERAN OR SPOUSE HAD MISCARRIAGES BEFORE PERSIAN GULF? ENTER ONE OF THE FOLLOWING CODES IN BLOCK 243. IF NO, GO TO ITEM 22D2.	Y=YES N=NO	(243)
22D1(a). STATE MATERNAL AGE AT CONCEPTION. ENTER AGE IN BLOCKS 244 AND 245.		(244) (245)
22D2. HAS VETERAN OR SPOUSE HAD MISCARRIAGES AFTER PERSIAN GULF? ENTER ONE OF THE FOLLOWING CODES IN BLOCK 246. IF NO, GO TO ITEM 22E.	Y=YES N=NO	(246)
22D2(a). STATE MATERNAL AGE AT CONCEPTION, ENTER AGE IN BLOCKS 247 AND 248.		(247) (248)
22E. HAS VETERAN OR SPOUSE HAD STILL BIRTH(S)? (NOTE: STILL BIRTH IS BIRTH AFTER 20 WEEKS OF GESTATION OF AN INFANT WHO SHOWED NO EVIDENCE OF LIFE AFTER BIRTH.) ENTER ONE OF THE FOLLOWING CODES IN BLOCK 249. IF NO, GO TO ITEM 22F.	Y=YES N=NO	(249)
22E1. HAS VETERAN OR SPOUSE HAD STILL BIRTH(S) BEFORE GULF SERVICE? ENTER ONE OF THE FOLLOWING CODES IN BLOCK 250. IF NO, GO TO ITEM 22E2.	Y=YES N=NO	(250)
22E1(a). STATE MATERNAL AGE AT CONCEPTION. ENTER AGE IN BLOCKS 251 AND 252.		(251) (252)
22E2. HAS VETERAN OR SPOUSE HAD STILL BIRTH(S) AFTER RETURN FROM GULF SERVICE? ENTER ONE OF THE FOLLOWING CODES IN BLOCK 253. IF NO, GO TO ITEM 22F.	Y=YES N=NO	(253)
22E2(a). STATE MATERNAL AGE AT CONCEPTION. ENTER AGE IN BLOCKS 254 AND 255.		(254) (255)
22F. HAS VETERAN OR SPOUSE HAD INFANT DEATH(S). (NOTE: DEATH THAT OCCURRED WITHIN ONE YEAR OF BIRTH AMONG BABIES BORN ALIVE.) ENTER ONE OF THE FOLLOWING CODES IN BLOCK 256. IF NO, GO TO ITEM 22G.	Y=YES N=NO	(256)
22F1. HAS VETERAN OR SPOUSE HAD INFANT DEATH(S) BEFORE GULF SERVICE? ENTER ONE OF THE FOLLOWING CODES IN BLOCK 257. IF NO, GO TO ITEM 22F2.	Y=YES N=NO	(257)
22F1(a). STATE MATERNAL AGE AT CONCEPTION. ENTER AGE IN BLOCKS 258 AND 259.		(258) (259)
22F2. HAS VETERAN OR SPOUSE HAD INFANT DEATH(S) AFTER GULF SERVICE ENTER ONE OF THE FOLLOWING CODES IN BLOCK 260. IF NO, GO TO ITEM 22G.	Y=YES N=NO	(260)

NAME: ____________________

SSN: ____________________

22F2(A) STATE MATERNAL AGE AT CONCEPTION. ENTER AGE IN BLOCKS 261 AND 262.	(261-262)

22G IF A WOMAN VETERAN REPORTS SHE WAS PREGNANT IN PERSIAN GULF, RECORD DATE OF CHILD'S BIRTH AND HOSPITAL OF BIRTH HERE AND IN VETERAN'S CHR ONLY TO FACILITATE FOLLOW-UP, IF NEEDED. (AAC WILL NOT ENTER THIS DATA IN PGR DATABASE).

DATE OF BIRTH ____________________ MONTH / DAY / YEAR

NAME OF HOSPITAL ____________________

LOCATION ____________________

PART II TO BE COMPLETED BY EXAMINING PHYSICIAN

23. DATE OF EXAM		
MONTH	DAY	YEAR
(263-264)	(265-266)	(267-270)

24. TOTAL NO. OF VETERAN'S COMPLAINTS.	(271-272)

25A/J. LIST UP TO TEN MAJOR, CURRENT SYMPTOMS, ICD 9 CODES, MO. & YR OF ONSET, DURATION IN MOS AND IF SYMPTOM IS CURRENTLY PRESENT ON LINES A-J, ITEMS 1-5. IF VETERAN HAS MORE THAN 10, ENTER THE MOST SEVERE & ADDITIONAL SYMPTOMS IN CHR. MAS CODERS: USE ITEM 2, BLOCKS 271-320 FOR ICD-9-CM CODES.

(1) DESCRIBE SYMPTOM NARRATIVE	(2) ICD-9-CODES (273-322)	(3) MO. & YR OF ONSET MONTH YEAR (323-382)	(4) DURATION (MONTHS) (383-402)	(5) CURRENTLY PRESENT? Y=Yes N=NO (403-412)
A	(273-277)	(323-328)	(383-384)	(403)
B	(278-282)	(329-334)	(385-386)	(404)
C	(283-287)	(335-340)	(387-388)	(405)
D	(288-292)	(341-346)	(389-390)	(406)
E	(293-297)	(347-352)	(391-392)	(407)
F	(298-302)	(353-358)	(393-394)	(408)
G	(303-307)	(359-364)	(395-396)	(409)
H	(308-312)	(365-370)	(397-398)	(410)
I	(313-317)	(371-376)	(399-400)	(411)
J	(318-322)	(377-382)	(401-402)	(412)

25K. LIST MOST SEVERE SYMPTOM. (A SYMPTOM FROM ITEM A-J, WHICH VETERAN CONSIDERS THE MOST SEVERE I.E. CHIEF COMPLAINT). ENTER ICD-9-CM CODE IN BLOCKS.	(413-417)

26. DIAGNOSTIC CONSULTATION. ENTER THE FOLLOWING CODES IN BLOCKS 418-435.

1=NO WORKUP. NO CONSULTATION DONE. 3=WORKUP/CONSULTATION DONE. DIAGNOSIS ESTABLISHED.

2=WORKUP/CONSULTATION DONE. UNEXPLAINED ILLNESS 4=WORKUP/CONSULTATION DONE. NO DIAGNOSIS.

A. ALLERGY/IMMUNOLOGY. BLOCK 418	(418)
B. AUDIOLOGY. BLOCK 419	(419)
C. CARDIOLOGY. BLOCK 420	(420)
D. DENTISTRY. BLOCK 421	(421)
E. DERMATOLOGY. BLOCK 422	(422)
F. EAR, NOSE AND THROAT 423	(423)
G. ENDOCRINOLOGY. BLOCK 424	(424)
H. GASTROENTEROLOGY. BLOCK 425	(425)

NAME: ____________________
SSN: ____________________

I. HEMATOLOGY/ONCOLOGY. BLOCK 426	(426)
J. INFECTIOUS DISEASES/PARASITOLOGY. BLOCK 427	(427)
K. NEPHROLOGY. BLOCK 428	(428)
L. NEUROLOGY. BLOCK 429	(429)
M. OCCUPATIONAL MEDICINE. BLOCK 430	(430)
N. PULMONARY. BLOCK 431	(431)
O. PSYCHIATRY. BLOCK 432	(432)
P. PSYCHOLOGY/PSYCHOMETRIC TESTING. BLOCK 433	(433)
Q. RHEUMATOLOGY. BLOCK 434	(434)
R. OTHER, ENTER FOLLOWING CODES IN BLOCK 435 Y=YES N=NO	(435)

S. ADDITIONAL WORKUPS/CONSULTATIONS PERFORMED WHICH WERE NOT LISTED IN ITEMS 26A-Q. LIST HERE AND IN CHR.

NAME: ____________________

SSN: ____________________

27. DIAGNOSIS. LIST UP TO 10 MAJOR DEFINITE MEDICAL DIAGNOSES ON LINES 27A-J. LIST PRIMARY DIAGNOSIS ON LINE A. BLOCKS 436-485 FOR CORRESPONDENCE ICD-9-CM CODES. LEAVE BLANK IF NO DIAGNOSIS IS MADE. MAS CODERS: USE ICD-9-CM CODES IN FIRST FIVE NUMBERED BLOCKS OF EACH DIAGNOSIS

27A. DESCRIBE DIAGNOSIS (Narrative)	(27B) ICD-9-CM (Codes)				
A. (PRIMARY)	(436)	(437)	(438)	(439)	(440)
B.	(441)	(442)	(443)	(444)	(445)
C.	(446)	(447)	(448)	(449)	(450)
D.	(451)	(452)	(453)	(454)	(455)
E.	(456)	(457)	(458)	(459)	(460)
F.	(461)	(462)	(463)	(464)	(465)
G.	(466)	(467)	(468)	(469)	(470)
H.	(471)	(472)	(473)	(474)	(475)
I.	(476)	(477)	(478)	(479)	(480)
J.	(481)	(482)	(483)	(484)	(485)

NOTE: CODERS: DO NOT REPEAT OR LIST SYMPTOM CODE ALREADY LISTED UNDER ITEM 25A-J.

28. BLOCK 486 IF NO DIAGNOSIS IS MADE, ENTER "1" IN BLOCK AT RIGHT, OTHERWISE, LEAVE BLANK. THIS ITEM MUST BE CONSIDERED IN CONJUNCTION WITH ITEM 27 "DIAGNOSIS." — 486

29. DISPOSITION (Enter code Y-Yes or N-No)

	Block		Block		Block
29A. EXAMINATION COMPLETED? Y=Yes N=No	487	29B. HOSPITALIZED AT VAMC FOR FURTHER TESTS? Y=Yes N=No	488	29C. HOSPITALIZED AT VAMC FOR TREATMENT? Y=Yes N=No	489
29D. REFERRED FOR OUTPATIENT CARE? Y=Yes N=No	490	29E. REFERRED TO PRIVATE PHYSICIAN, NON-VA CLINIC OR NON-VA HOSPITAL? Y=Yes N=No	491	29F. BIOPSY? Y=Yes N=No	492

	Block		Block
30. AFTER COMPLETION OF PHASE I EXAM (REFER TO PAR 5), THE PHYSICIAN HAS DETERMINED THE VETERAN HAS UNEXPLAINED ILLNESS? Y=Yes N=No	493	31. HAS PHASE II EXAM (REFER TO CH. 3) BEEN INITIATED? Y=Yes N=No	494

32. UTILIZE THIS SECTION FOR ADDITIONAL INFORMATION (E.G. PAR 1.07 - M-10, PT III).

33. NAME OF EXAMINER. (PRINT FULL NAME)

34. TITLE OF EXAMINER. (FULL TITLE OF EXAMINER)

35. SIGNATURE OF EXAMINER.

35A. SIGNATURE OF VRP (VETERANS REGISTRY PHYSICIAN)

NAME: ____________________

SSN: ____________________

PART III

PHASE II - UNIFORM CASE ASSESSMENT (UCA)

1. WERE THE FOLLOWING TESTS PERFORMED? Enter the following codes in blocks 1-24. Y = YES N = NO
2. BLOOD TESTS. BLOCKS 1-18; OTHER - BLOCKS 19-24.

A. CBC (COMPLETE BLOOD COUNT)	(1)	B. SED RATE? (SKIN ERETHYMA DOSE)	(2)	C. C-REACTIVE PROTEIN	(3)
D. RHEMATOID FACTOR?	(4)	E. FLUORESCENT ANA? (ANTI-NUCLEAR ANTI-BODY)	(5)	F. SGOT (AST)? (GLUTAMIC OXALOACETIC TRANSAMINASE)	(6)
G. SGPT (ALT) (TRANSAMINASE GLUTAMIC PYRUVATE)	(7)	H. LDH (LACTIC ACID HYDROGENASE)	(8)	I. ALKALINE PHOSPHATASE	(9)
J. CPK? CREATINE PHOSPHOKINASE)	(10)	K. HEPATITIS B SURFACE ANTIBODY?	(11)	L. HEPATITIS B CORE ANTIGEN?	(12)
M. VDRL? (VENEREAL DISEASE RESEARCH LABORATORY)	(13)	N. VITAMIN B-12	(14)	O. FOLATE?	(15)
P. HIV (HUMAN IMMUNO-DEFICIENCY)	(16)	Q. T4 (THROXINE TOTAL SERUM)?	(17)	R. TSH (THYROID STIMULATING HORMONE)?	(18)
3. URINALYSIS	(19)	4. TB SKIN TEST (PPD)? (TUBERCULOSIS SKIN TEST PURIFIED PROTEIN DERIVATIVE)	(20)	5. CHEST XRAY	(21)
6. PSYCHIATRIC EVALUATION?	(22)	6A. SCID FOR DSM-III-R (STRUCTURED CLINICAL INTERVIEW FOR DIAGNOSIS)	(23)	6B. CAPS PTSD SCALE (CLINICAL ADMINISTERED POST TRAUMATIC STRESS DISORDER)	(24)

7. LIST DIAGNOSES: MAS CODERS: ENTER ICD-9-CM CODE IN BLOCKS 25-39. IF NONE, LEAVE BLANK.

DESCRIBE DIAGNOSES (Narrative)	ICD-9-CODES				
1.	(25)	(26)	(27)	(28)	(29)
2.	(30)	(31)	(32)	(33)	(34)
3.	(35)	(36)	(37)	(38)	(39)

8. PSYCHOLOGY-NEUROPSYCHOLOGICAL TEST? Enter code in block 40) (40)

Y=Yes N=No

8A. LIST DIAGNOSES. MAS CODERS: ENTER ICD-9-CM CODES IN BLOCKS 41-55. IF NONE, LEAVE BLANK

DESCRIBE DIAGNOSES (Narrative)	ICD-9-CODES				
1.	(41)	(42)	(43)	(44)	(45)
2.	(46)	(47)	(48)	(49)	(50)
3.	(51)	(52)	(53)	(54)	(55)

9. INFECTIOUS DISEASE - SCREENING EXAM? (Enter code in block 56) (56)

Y=Yes N=No

9A. LIST DIAGNOSES. MAS CODERS: ENTER ICD-9-CM CODES IN BLOCKS 57-66. IF NONE, LEAVE BLANK

DESCRIBE DIAGNOSES (Narrative)	ICD-9-CODES				
1.	(57)	(58)	(59)	(60)	(61)
2.	(62)	(63)	(64)	(65)	(66)

10. DENTAL EXAM? (Enter code in block 67) (67)

Y=Yes N=No

10A. LIST DIAGNOSES. MAS CODERS: ENTER ICD-9-CM CODES IN BLOCKS 68-77. IF NONE, LEAVE BLANK

DESCRIBE DIAGNOSES (Narrative)	ICD-9-CODES				
1.	(68)	(69)	(70)	(71)	(72)
2.	(73)	(74)	(75)	(76)	(77)

NAME: ____________________

SSN: ____________________

11. DIARRHEA AND/OR ABDOMINAL PAIN

11A. GI (GASTROINTESTINAL) CONSULT? (Enter code in block 78) Y = Yes N = No	78	11B. LIST DIAGNOSES. MAS CODERS: ENTER ICD-9-CM CODES IN BLOCKS 79-98. IF NONE, LEAVE BLANK.					
		DESCRIBE DIAGNOSES (Narrative)	ICD-9-CODES				
		1.	(79)	(80)	(81)	(82)	(83)
		2.	(84)	(85)	(86)	(87)	(88)
		3.	(89)	(90)	(91)	(92)	(93)
		4.	(94)	(95)	(96)	(97)	(98)

12. HEADACHE AND/OR MEMORY LOSS

12A. NEUROLOGY CONSULT? (Enter code in block 99) Y = Yes N = No	99	12B. LIST DIAGNOSES. MAS CODERS: ENTER ICD-9-CM CODES IN BLOCKS 100-109. IF NONE, LEAVE BLANK.					
		DESCRIBE DIAGNOSES (Narrative)	ICD-9-CODES				
		1.	(100)	(101)	(102)	(103)	(104)
		2.	(105)	(106)	(107)	(108)	(109)

13. MUSCLE ACHES AND/OR NUMBNESS

13A. NEUROLOGY CONSULT? (Enter code in block 110) Y = Yes N = No	110	13B. LIST DIAGNOSES. MAS CODERS: ENTER ICD-9-CM CODES IN BLOCKS 111-120. IF NONE, LEAVE BLANK.					
		DESCRIBE DIAGNOSES (Narrative)	ICD-9-CODES				
		1.	(111)	(112)	(113)	(114)	(115)
		2.	(116)	(117)	(118)	(119)	(120)

14. CHRONIC FATIGUE

14A. CHRONIC FATIGUE? (Enter code in block 121) Y = Yes N = No	121	14B. LIST DIAGNOSES. MAS CODERS: ENTER ICD-9-CM CODES IN BLOCKS 122-131. IF NONE, LEAVE BLANK.					
		DESCRIBE DIAGNOSES (Narrative)	ICD-9-CODES				
		1.	(122)	(123)	(124)	(125)	(126)
		2.	(127)	(128)	(129)	(130)	(131)

15. JOINT PAIN

15A. RHEUMATOLOGY CONSULT? (Enter code in block 132) Y = Yes N = No	132	15B. LIST DIAGNOSES. MAS CODERS: ENTER ICD-9-CM CODES IN BLOCKS 133-142. IF NONE, LEAVE BLANK.					
		DESCRIBE DIAGNOSES (Narrative)	ICD-9-CODES				
		1.	(133)	(134)	(135)	(136)	(137)
		2.	(138)	(139)	(140)	(141)	(142)

16. CHRONIC COUGH AND/OR SHORTNESS OF BREATH

16A. PULMONARY CONSULT? (Enter code in block 143) Y = Yes N = No	143	16B. LIST DIAGNOSES. MAS CODERS: ENTER ICD-9-CM CODES IN BLOCKS 144-153. IF NONE, LEAVE BLANK.					
		DESCRIBE DIAGNOSES (Narrative)	ICD-9-CODES				
		1.	(144)	(145)	(146)	(147)	(158)
		2.	(149)	(150)	(151)	(152)	(153)

17. SKIN RASH

17A. DERMATOLOGY CONSULT? (Enter code in block 154) Y = Yes N = No	154	17B. LIST DIAGNOSES. MAS CODERS: ENTER ICD-9-CM CODES IN BLOCKS 155-164. IF NONE, LEAVE BLANK.					
		DESCRIBE DIAGNOSES (Narrative)	ICD-9-CODES				
		1.	(155)	(156)	(157)	(158)	(159)
		2.	(160)	(161)	(162)	(163)	(164)

18. VERTIGO AND/OR TINNITUS

18A. AUDIOLOGY? (Enter code in block 165) Y = Yes N = No	165	18B. LIST DIAGNOSES. MAS CODERS: ENTER ICD-9-CM CODES IN BLOCKS 166-175. IF NONE, LEAVE BLANK.					
		DESCRIBE DIAGNOSES (Narrative)	ICD-9-CODES				
		1.	(166)	(167)	(168)	(169)	(170)
		2.	(171)	(172)	(173)	(174)	(175)

NAME: ____________________

SSN: ____________________

19. CHEST PAIN AND/OR PALPITATIONS

19A. CARDIOLOGY CONSULT (Enter code in block 176) Y=YES N=NO	176	19B. LIST DIAGNOSES. MAS CODERS ENTER ICD-9-CM CODES IN BLOCKS 177-186. IF NONE, LEAVE BLANK					
		DESCRIBE DIAGNOSES (Narrative)	ICD-9-CODES				
		1.	(177)	(178)	(179)	(180)	(181)
		2.	(182)	(183)	(184)	(185)	(186)

20. REPRODUCTIVE CONCERNS

20A. MALES - UROLOGY CONSULT? (Enter code in block 187) Y=YES N=NO	187	188. LIST DIAGNOSES. MAS CODERS ENTER ICD-9-CM CODES IN BLOCKS 189-198. IF NONE, LEAVE BLANK					
		DESCRIBE DIAGNOSES (Narrative)	ICD-9-CODES				
20B. FEMALES - GYN CONSULT? (Enter code in block 188) Y=YES N=NO	188	1.	(189)	(190)	(191)	(192)	(193)
		2.	(194)	(195)	(196)	(197)	(198)

21. FINAL DIAGNOSES: PHASES II

21A. DIAGNOSES. LIST UP TO 10 MAJOR DEFINITE MEDICAL DIAGNOSES ON LINES 20A-J. LIST PRIMARY DIAGNOSIS ON LINE A. BLOCKS 199-248 OR CORRESPONDING ICD-9-CM CODES. LEAVE BLANK IF NO DIAGNOSIS IS MADE. MAS CODERS: USE ICD-9-CM CODES IN FIRST FIVE NUMBERED BLOCKS OF EACH DIAGNOSIS

DESCRIBE DIAGNOSES (Narrative)	ICD-9-CODES				
A. (PRIMARY)	(199)	(200)	(201)	(202)	(203)
B.	(204)	(205)	(206)	(207)	(208)
C.	(209)	(210)	(211)	(212)	(213)
D.	(214)	(215)	(216)	(217)	(218)
E.	(219)	(220)	(221)	(222)	(223)
F.	(224)	(225)	(226)	(227)	(228)
G.	(229)	(230)	(231)	(232)	(233)
H.	(234)	(235)	(236)	(237)	(238)
I.	(239)	(240)	(241)	(242)	(243)
J.	(244)	(245)	(246)	(247)	(248)

22. AFTER COMPLETING PHASE II, UNIFORM CASE ASSESSMENT PROTOCOL, THE PHYSICIAN FEELS THAT THE VETERAN HAS AN UNEXPLAINED ILLNESS? (Enter code in block 249) Y=YES N=NO	(249)

Appendix I

VA Persian Gulf Bi-Monthly Report

INSTRUCTIONS AND SAMPLE FORMAT FOR COMPLETION OF BI-MONTHLY REPORT ON PERSIAN GULF WAR VETERANS REGISTRY EXAMINATIONS (RCS 10-0860)

A bi-monthly report is required from all Department of Veterans Affairs (VA) facilities providing up-to-date statistical information on Persian Gulf Registry (PGR) examinations. Instructions are provided below for the completion and submission of this report.

1. Date of Report. Each report should include the date the report was prepared and submitted to the following address:

2. Mailing Address. This report should be transmitted to the following address:

Department of Veterans Affairs
Environmental Agents Service (131)
ATTN: Persian Gulf Coordinator
810 Vermont Avenue, N.W.
Washington, DC 20420

3. Mailing Date. This report should be sent to the above address NO LATER THAN 5 WORKING DAYS FOLLOWING THE END OF EACH BI-MONTHLY REPORTING PERIOD.

4. The following statistical information is required (see sample 2F-3 and 2F-4).

a. Initial Examination. (The first physical examination of the Persian Gulf veteran.) List the total number of completed initial examinations performed during the current 2-month reporting period. *NOTE: A completed code sheet has already been sent to Austin Automation Center (AAC) which was completed for the purpose of entering a Persian Gulf veteran into the PGR. This count should be verified with the computerized or card file records maintained at each facility (see par. 2.04) describing the computerized or card file requirement.*

b. Cumulative Initial Examinations. The total number of cumulative initial examinations listed in the previous bi-monthly report.

c. Cumulative Initial Examination. The total number of "first-time" examinations performed by the medical facility since the beginning of the PGR in 1992. This number should include the current month's initial examinations (par. 4a) plus the sum of the previous month's cumulative initial examinations (par. 4b). *NOTE: Examinations performed by satellite outpatient clinics should be included in the total cumulative figure for VA medical center of jurisdiction. Justification for exceptions to this requirement should be directed to EAS (131), VHA Headquarters. Independent outpatient clinics should report in a manner similar to VA medical centers.*

d. Initial Incomplete Examinations (in process). The total number of incomplete (code sheet(s) that has/have not been sent to AAC) initial examinations in process during the period of the current report.

e. Follow-up Examinations. (A first-time examination subsequent to the initial examination—a completed initial examination code sheet has been sent to AAC). The total number of follow-up examinations during the period of the current report.

f. Cumulative Follow-up Examinations. The total number of follow-up examinations performed by the medical facility since the beginning of the registry in 1992. This total should be the sum of the previous months' cumulative follow-up examination total and the current bi-monthly follow-up examinations.

g. Follow-up Examinations in Process. The total number of follow-up examinations being processed (completed code sheet(s) has/have not been sent to AAC).

h. Pending Examination Appointments. The total number of initial Persian Gulf examinations for which appointments have been scheduled beyond the end of the bi-monthly report period. *NOTE: This is not cumulative and applies to the current bi-monthly report.*

i. Next Appointment Date. Indicate the next available appointment date.

j. Number of Veterans Failing to Keep an Initial Examination Appointment. The total number of veterans who failed to keep a scheduled appointment during the bi-monthly reporting report. *NOTE: This is not cumulative and applies to reporting period only.*

k. Comments or Problems Regarding Pending Examination Appointments. Problems or challenges should be documented with comments regarding examination workload. An explanation and action plan to alleviate delays should be provided in situations where a facility has 50 or more examinations pending, and/or the next available appointment is more than 30 days beyond the date of request. If statistics have been adjusted due to AAC acceptance of code sheets, the message "Cumulative statistics adjusted per transaction acceptance at AAC" need to be included in this paragraph.

l. Name and Telephone Number: The name and telephone number of the person preparing the report must be indicated.

SAMPLE FORMAT FOR BI-MONTHLY REPORT ON PERSIAN GULF VETERANS (RCS-10-0860)

DEPARTMENT OF VETERANS AFFAIRS
Medical Center
Anywhere, USA 85012

In Reply Refer to:

August 7, 1995

Department of Veterans Affairs
Environmental Agents Service (131)
ATTN: Persian Gulf Coordinator
810 Vermont Avenue, N.W.
Washington, DC 20420

SUBJECT: Bi-monthly Report of Persian Gulf War Veteran Registry Examinations, (RCS-10-0860)—Period Ending July 31, 1995 (Station #600)

The subject report is submitted for the 2-month period ending July 31, 1995:

a. Initial Examination (Current Bi-Monthly Reporting Period):
List total number of completed initial examinations performed for 2-month period ending July 31, 1995 (i.e., total number of Persian Gulf Registry code sheets submitted to Austin Automation Center (AAC): 100

b. Cumulative Initial Examinations from Previous Bi-Monthly Report: +450

c. Cumulative Number of Completed Initial Examinations Performed Since Onset of Program (August, 1992):
Total of numbers listed in Paragraphs 1-a and 1-b 550

Note: This should be the total number of all initial examination code sheets submitted to AAC since onset of program. If code sheets have not been sent to AAC, do not include in this total.

d. Initial Incomplete Examinations (in process);
Total number of initial (incomplete examinations in process: (code sheets have not been sent to AAC): 75

e. Follow-Up Examinations (Code Sheets Sent to AAC):
Total number of follow-up examinations performed for current reporting period (follow-up examinations are those performed subsequent to the initial examination where a completed code sheet for an initial examination has been sent to AAC): 15

f. Cumulative Follow-up Examinations:
Includes the total of follow-up examinations performed (this total includes the number listed in above (par. 1-e) and all follow-up examinations previously reported since August, 1992). 75

g. Follow-up Examinations in Process:
Total number of follow-up examinations in process (code sheets have not been sent to AAC during this reporting period): 12

h. Pending Examination Appointments:
Total number of initial examinations for which appointments have been scheduled beyond the end of the bi-monthly report period: 20

i. The Next Available Appointment Date: 8/10/95

j. Number of Veterans Failing to Keep an Initial Examination Appointment:
Total number of veterans who failed to keep a scheduled appointment during the current bi-monthly reporting period. This is not cumulative. 10

k. Comments/problems regarding pending examinations: None

l. The name, address and telephone number of the person preparing this report:

(Signature)
John Doe
Medical Center Director

Appendix J

Examples of Persian Gulf Registry Follow-Up Letters

SAMPLE PERSIAN GULF VETERANS FOLLOW-UP LETTER (MEDICAL PROBLEMS INDICATED)

DEPARTMENT OF VETERANS AFFAIRS
Medical Center
Anywhere, USA 85012

In Reply Refer to:

(Date)

(Name/Address)

Dear ______________________:

We sincerely appreciate your recent participation in the Department of Veterans Affairs (VA) Persian Gulf Registry. This effort should prove to be helpful in assisting us to serve you and other veterans who are concerned about the possible health problems which may have resulted from service in Southwest Asia during the Persian Gulf War.

As discussed at the conclusion of your visit, results of your examination and laboratory tests showed certain problems (optional—these findings may be described in lay terms). In view of these findings, we have scheduled you for treatment of these health problems on **(date)**. If for any reason you cannot keep this appointment, please call (**telephone number**) at the earliest possible time to cancel and reschedule.

The results of your examination will be maintained by VA and will be available for future use as needed. If you have any questions or concerns about your Persian Gulf Registry examination, please contact the Veterans' Registry Coordinator at (**telephone number**) for assistance.

Whether you are entitled to cost-free treatment or will be responsible for partial co-payment will be determined by your income and other factors unless the VA determines that your health problems are service connected. You may wish to file a claim for compensation to establish possible service connection. The injury or illness need not have been incurred in combat; the law requires only that a disease or disability was incurred or aggravated during military service.

Please remember that this examination does not automatically initiate a claim for VA benefits. If you wish to file a claim, please contact your nearest VA Regional Office. In your area the Regional Office is located at (**address**). Their telephone number is (**telephone number**). If you need any further assistance, you may contact a Veterans' Benefits Counselor by calling the VA toll-free telephone number 1-800-827-1000.

An outreach program has been implemented by which VA notifies all individuals listed in the Registry of significant VA activities, including the health consequences of military service in the Persian Gulf theater of operations during the Persian Gulf War. You will be receiving a "Persian Gulf Review" which is published periodically by VA's Environmental Agents Service. A copy of this "Review" is enclosed for your reference.

We trust this information is helpful to you. Once again, your participation in the registry is appreciated.

Sincerely,

(Signature)

Name of Veterans' Registry Physician

Enclosure

SAMPLE PERSIAN GULF VETERANS FOLLOW-UP LETTER (NO MEDICAL PROBLEMS INDICATED)

DEPARTMENT OF VETERANS AFFAIRS
Medical Center
Anywhere, USA 85012

In Response Reply Refer to:

(Date)

(Name/Address)

Dear ______________________:

We sincerely appreciate your recent participation in the Department of Veterans Affairs (VA) Persian Gulf Registry. This effort should prove to be helpful in assisting us to serve you and other veterans who are concerned about the possible health problems which may have resulted from service in Southwest Asia during the Persian Gulf War.

As discussed at the conclusion of your visit, results of your examination and laboratory tests indicate that there are no detectable medical problems. At this time you have no reason to be concerned about any adverse health effects resulting from your service in the Persian Gulf. However, in the future if you have a medical problem, I would encourage you to seek the help and advice of your nearest VA medical center or outpatient clinic. You may reach us at **(telephone number)**.

The results of your examination will be maintained by VA and will be available for future use as needed.

Please remember that this examination does not automatically initiate a claim for VA benefits. If you wish to file a claim, please contact your nearest VA Regional Office. In your area the Regional Office is located at (**address**). Their telephone number is (**telephone number**). If you need any further assistance, you may contact a Veterans' Benefits Counselor by calling the VA toll-free telephone number 1-800-827-1000.

An outreach program has been implemented by which VA notifies all individuals listed in the Registry of significant VA activities, including the health consequences of military service in the Persian Gulf theater of operations during the Persian Gulf War. You will be receiving a "Persian Gulf Review" which is published periodically by VA's Environmental Agents Service. A copy of this "Review" is enclosed for your reference.

We trust this information is helpful to you. Once again, your participation in the registry is appreciated.

Sincerely,

(Signature)
Name of Veterans' Registry Physician

Enclosure

Appendix K

VA Monitoring Instrument for Appropriate Medical Care

VHA DIRECTIVE 96-051 (August 14, 1996)
PERSIAN GULF VETERANS

The mission of the Persian Gulf (PG) Veterans Program is to provide strategic direction for the clinical, research, education and outreach programs for PG veterans. This is accomplished by working in collaboration with other VA offices; Federal, state, and local government agencies; and nonprofit community and private providers. The Persian Gulf Veterans Program also serves as VHA's liaison to the Persian Gulf Veterans Interagency Coordinating Board.

Population Measures

1. Waiting time for appointment for Registry examination and referral center admission.
   GOAL: ≤30 days in 95% of VAMCs

2. Education
   a. Provide opportunities for continuing medical education of Persian Gulf War (PGW) health issues
   GOAL: National Training Program
   (1) Onsite conference (8/27–8/28)
   (2) Teleconferences (satellite video broadcasts) Two in 1996

   b. Provide current information on PGW programs, legislation, reports and publications.

GOAL: Quarterly mailouts and newsletter, periodic Environmental Agents Services (EAS) conference calls

3. Future—PGW veteran satisfaction with VA healthcare.
GOAL: Satisfaction ≥ other veteran groups

Program Measures

1. Waiting times for appointments for consultations, e.g., neurology, rheumatology, gastroenterology, psychiatry, psychology, etc.
GOAL: =<45 days

2. Persian Gulf Registry: Phase I and Phase II code sheets rejection rates
GOAL: rate=<5%

3. Time to correct rejected code sheets
GOAL: =<30 DAYS

4. Compliance threshold on the annual Quality Management monitor for Persian Gulf Registry Examinations as measured against selected clinical indicators
GOAL: 90%

5. Participation rates of Persian Gulf Coordinators and Registry Physicians in information and educational activities, i.e., quarterly Environmental Agents Service conference calls, satellite video-television broadcasts, and continuing medical education conference
GOAL: 75%

VHA DIRECTIVE 10-95-114 (November 21, 1995) PERSIAN GULF REGISTRY HEALTH EXAMINATION PROGRAM QUALITY MANAGEMENT/SELF ASSESSMENT MONITOR (RCS 10-0860)

1. **PURPOSE**: The purpose of this Veterans Health Administration (VHA) Directive is to provide procedures on use of VA Form 10-9009C-1, Persian Gulf Registry Health Examination Program—Quality Management/Self Assessment Monitor (Att.). This instrument has been developed as a quality management tool for conducting reviews of Persian Gulf War veteran's medical records. It is to be used by VA medical centers to assess and monitor the appropriateness of medical care being provided in accordance with the Protocol for conducting the

Physical Examination and Ordering Diagnostic Studies (M-10, Pt. III, Ch. 2, App. 2B).

2. **BACKGROUND**: Approximately 697,000 American servicemen and service women were involved in the Persian Gulf War. A number of these troops may have been exposed to environmental hazards, and/or possible diseases endemic to the Southwest Asia theater of operation.

a. Public Law 102-585, enacted in November 1992, authorized establishment of the VA's Persian Gulf War Veterans Health Registry. That law authorized the VA to provide a comprehensive medical examination, including any diagnostic testing, to evaluate the veteran's health status.

b. An Office of Inspector General (OIG) Report, "An Oversight Evaluation of the Department of Veterans Affairs' Response to Health Care Issues Relating to Military Service in the Persian Gulf War" (5HI-A28-011; December 29, 1994), recommended that VA facilities assure that all Persian Gulf War veterans have been afforded appropriate medical care by conducting peer reviews of a statistically valid sample of Gulf veteran's medical records.

3. **POLICY**: VA is committed to providing high quality medical care to veterans, and to ensure that this goal is met for Persian Gulf War veterans, appropriate mechanisms must be put in place to address their special needs and health problems. We also must monitor the effectiveness of the services provided to them.

4. **ACTION**

a. Each VA medical center will use the Persian Gulf Registry Health Examination Program—Quality Management/Self Assessment Monitor to review, at least, a 10% sample of all Persian Gulf Registry physical examinations conducted to date.

b. The first such review will be conducted by each VA medical center within a time-frame that ensures that results are provided to the Environmental Agents Program (131), VHA Headquarters, no later than January 31, 1996. Subsequent reviews should be conducted on an annual basis thereafter, with results submitted to (131) by October 1 of each year.

c. Results of the review should be recorded on VA Form 10-9009C-2, Summary Analysis of Self Assessment Monitor Results (Att. B) for submission at the following address:

Director, Environmental Agents Program (131)
VHA Headquarters
810 Vermont Avenue, N.W.
Washington, DC 20420
FAX 202-565-7572

d. Questions may be referred to Director, Environmental Agents Program (131), at 202-565-4183, or Environmental Agents Program staff at 202-565-4548.

5. **REFERENCES**

a. M-10, Part III, Chapters 1–4

b. Office of Inspector General (OIG) Report, "An Oversight Evaluation of the Department of Veterans Affairs' Response to Health Care Issues Relating to Military Service in the Persian Gulf War" (5HI-A28-011; December 29, 1994).

6. **FOLLOW-UP RESPONSIBILITY**: Director, Environmental Agents Program (131), is responsible for the content of this Directive.

7. **RECISSIONS**: None. This VHA Directive will expire November 21, 2000.

Kenneth W. Kizer, M.D., M.P.H.
Under Secretary for Health

Attachments

ATTACHMENT A

PERSIAN GULF REGISTRY HEALTH EXAMINATION QUALITY MANAGEMENT/SELF ASSESSMENT MONITOR

FACILITY LOCATION (City & State): ____________________
FACILITY NUMBER: ____________________
PERSIAN GULF COORDINATOR: ____________________
VETERANS REGISTRY PHYSICIAN(S): ____________________

PATIENT NAME (LAST/FIRST/MI): ____________________

PATIENT SSN:
☐☐☐ - ☐☐ - ☐☐☐☐

A. Required Components of the Registry Examination

	Yes	No	Refused
Code Sheet in CHR Consolidated Health Record	☐	☐	
1. Thorough History and Physical Examination in CHR, such as completion of an SF88	☐	☐	
2. Women Persian Gulf Veterans			
a. Breast Exam	☐	☐	☐
b. Gynecology Exam	☐	☐	☐
3. Laboratory Results in CHR:			
a. CBC	☐	☐	
b. Chemistries	☐	☐	
c. Urinalysis	☐	☐	

d. Chest x-ray — Yes ☐ No ☐

4. A follow-up visit is recorded? — Yes ☐ No ☐ NA ☐

5. Follow-up letter, containing exam results and recommendations is in CHR (or mailed)? — Yes ☐ No ☐

6. Additional Diagnostic Work-up for Selected Symptoms:

The following examinations were ordered by the physician, if the veteran complained of:

a. Persistent Diarrhea

i. Rectal Exam — Yes ☐ No ☐ Refused ☐

ii. Stool guaiac — Yes ☐ No ☐

iii. Stool WBC — Yes ☐ No ☐

iv. Stool for ova/parasite — Yes ☐ No ☐

v. GI consult — Yes ☐ No ☐

b. Memory Loss

i. Mini-Mental Status Exam or other bedside memory test — Yes ☐ No ☐

ii. Additional Labs:

Thyroid function — Yes ☐ No ☐

VDRL (RPR) Yes ☐ No ☐

B12 Yes ☐ No ☐

Other (Neurology consult, CT/MRI) Yes ☐ No ☐

c. Shortness of Breath or Chronic Cough

i. Lung Exam Recorded Yes ☐ No ☐

ii. Pulmonary Function Test Yes ☐ No ☐

iii. Smoking History Yes ☐ No ☐

B. Follow-up Appointments

1. If the veteran was symptomatic at the time of completion of the Registry exam was a follow-up examination scheduled? Yes ☐ No ☐

2. Has the veteran been assigned to a primary care team? Yes ☐ No ☐

ATTACHMENT B

SUMMARY ANALYSIS OF SELF-ASSESSMENT MONITOR RESULTS

VAMC/OPC: CITY STATE:

VAMC/OPC NUMBER: VISN SITE NUMBER:

PERSON COMPLETING SURVEY:

LAST NAME: FIRST NAME:

TELEPHONE NUMBER:

AREA CODE - - EXTENSION

A. BACKGROUND:

1) NUMBER OF PERSIAN GULF VETERANS WHO RECEIVED REGISTRY EXAMINATIONS IN 19____ (STATE YEAR). N =

2) SAMPLE PERCENTAGE = %

% Male % Female

B. STANDARD REGISTRY EXAM:

1) NUMBER OF CHARTS THAT CONTAINED CODE SHEETS N =

NON-COMPLIANCE = %

2) NUMBER OF CHARTS THAT CONTAINED A HISTORY AND PHYSICAL (SF88) N =

NON-COMPLIANCE = %

3) NUMBER OF CHARTS THAT CONTAINED CBC TEST RESULTS

N = ☐☐☐☐

NON-COMPLIANCE = ☐☐☐%

4) NUMBER OF CHARTS THAT CONTAINED CHEMISTRIES

N = ☐☐☐☐

NON-COMPLIANCE = ☐☐☐%

5) NUMBER OF CHARTS THAT CONTAINED URINALYSIS

N = ☐☐☐☐

NON-COMPLIANCE = ☐☐☐%

6) NUMBER OF CHARTS THAT CONTAINED CHEST X-RAY

N = ☐☐☐☐

NON-COMPLIANCE = ☐☐☐%

7) NUMBER OF CHARTS THAT RECORDED A FOLLOW-UP VISIT

N = ☐☐☐☐

NON-COMPLIANCE = ☐☐☐%

8) NUMBER OF CHARTS THAT CONTAINED A FOLLOW-UP LETTER

N = ☐☐☐☐

NON-COMPLIANCE = ☐☐☐%

C. WORK-UP FOR COMMON COMPLAINTS:

9) NUMBER OF CHARTS THAT CONTAINED SYMPTOM-SPECIFIC EXAMINATIONS IF PATIENT COMPLAINED OF PERSISTENT DIARRHEA

N = ☐☐☐☐

NON-COMPLIANCE = ☐☐☐%

10) NUMBER OF CHARTS THAT CONTAINED SYMPTOM-SPECIFIC EXAMINATIONS IF PATIENT COMPLAINED OF MEMORY LOSS

N = ☐☐☐☐

NON-COMPLIANCE = ☐☐☐%

11) NUMBER OF CHARTS THAT CONTAINED SYMPTOM-SPECIFIC EXAMINATIONS IF PATIENT COMPLAINED OF SHORTNESS OF BREATH/CHRONIC COUGH

N = ☐☐☐☐

NON-COMPLIANCE = ☐☐☐ %

12) NUMBER OF CHARTS THAT SHOWED A FOLLOW-UP APPOINTMENT HAD BEEN SCHEDULED

N = ☐☐☐☐

NON-COMPLIANCE = ☐☐☐ %

D. PRIMARY CARE TEAM ASSIGNMENT:

13) NUMBER OF CHARTS THAT SHOWED PATIENT HAD BEEN ASSIGNED TO A PRIMARY CARE TEAM

N = ☐☐☐☐

NON-COMPLIANCE = ☐☐☐ %

E. WOMEN VETERANS:

14) NUMBER OF FEMALE PATIENT CHARTS THAT SHOWED COMPLETION OF A BREAST EXAMINATION

N = ☐☐☐☐

NON-COMPLIANCE = ☐☐☐ %

15) NUMBER OF FEMALE PATIENT CHARTS THAT SHOWED COMPLETION OF GYNECOLOGY EXAMINATION

N = ☐☐☐☐

NON-COMPLIANCE = ☐☐☐ %

Appendix L

Annual Persian Gulf Conference Agenda

EMPLOYEE EDUCATION SYSTEM
ST. LOUIS EDUCATION CENTER

presents

COURSE NO. 97-NP

HEALTH CONSEQUENCES OF PERSIAN GULF SERVICE
JUNE 3–4, 1997

in cooperation with

THE OFFICE OF EMPLOYEE EDUCATION
OFFICE OF PUBLIC HEALTH AND ENVIRONMENTAL HAZARDS
AND
ENVIRONMENTAL AGENTS SERVICE
DEPARTMENT OF VETERANS AFFAIRS

PLACE Hyatt Regency, 200 South Pine Avenue, Long Beach, California

PURPOSE

This program is designed to provide an update on the latest information available from the clinical and scientific studies of Persian Gulf veterans' illnesses. It will focus on information needed to enhance clinical skills in the evaluation and management of Gulf War veterans.

OBJECTIVES

At the conclusion of this program, participants will be able to:

1. describe current Persian Gulf War (PGW) veterans' programs available through VA and British and Canadian military forces;

2. discuss the Presidential Advisory Committee's recommendations and government responses;

3. use the assessment, treatment, and communication approaches presented during the program in their work with PGW veterans;

4. provide a comprehensive Persian Gulf Veteran's program including occupational exposure assessments, clinical and C&P exams, and the management of special issues in the care of the PGW veteran;

5. include psychosocial aspects as a part of the assessment and treatment of the PGW veteran; and

6. apply relevant research studies' findings concerning Gulf War veterans' illnesses to their medical care and treatment.

EXPECTED OUTCOMES

Each participant will use the information presented to enhance the evaluation and treatment of PGW veterans.

TARGET AUDIENCE

This conference is designed for VA Medical Center Persian Gulf physicians and clinical staff and selected readjustment counseling staff. Additional participants will be selected by the Office of Public Health and Environmental Hazards on a space available basis.

PROGRAM SCHEDULE

Monday, June 2, 1997

6:00–8:00 pm	Registration	***Regency Ballroom Lobby***

Tuesday, June 3, 1997

Moderator: Frances M. Murphy, MD, MPH

7:00 am	Registration	***Regency Ballroom Lobby***

General Session ***Regency Ballroom***

8:00 Welcome
Susan Mather, MD

8:15 Update on VA PGW Programs
Frances M. Murphy, MD, MPH

8:45 Update on British PGW Programs
Col. Timothy P. Finnegan, MBBS, MSc, FFOM

9:15 Update on Canadian PGW Programs
Lt. Col. Kenneth C. Scott, MD

9:45 Break

10:15 Presidential Advisory Committee Report and Recommendations
Joyce C. Lashof, MD

10:45 Alternative Hypotheses for Causation of Persian Gulf War Veterans' Illnesses
Robert H. Roswell, MD

11:15 War Syndromes and Their Evaluation
Kenneth Craig Hyams, MD

11:45 Panel Discussion
Moderator: Frances M. Murphy, MD, MPH
Col. Timothy P. Finnegan, BSc, MBBS, MSc, FFOM
Kenneth Craig Hyams, MD
Joyce C. Lashof, MD

Robert H. Roswell, MD
Lt. Col. Kenneth C. Scott, MD

12:30 Lunch

1:30 *Concurrent Sessions*

1. Physiologic Effects of Traumatic and Non-Traumatic Stress ***Shoreline A/B***
Moderator: Theresa L. King, PA-C
Matthew J. Friedman, MD, PhD

2. The Tokyo Subway Incident of 20 March 1995 ***Regency Ballroom***
Moderator: Frances M. Murphy, MD, MPH
Annetta P. Watson, PhD

3. Health Risk Communication to Persian Gulf Veterans ***Harbor A/B/C***
Moderator: Donald J. Rosenblum, Max R. Lum, E.Ed., M.P.A.
Timothy L. Tinker, DrPH, MPH

4. Compensation and Pension Exams for Persian Gulf Veterans' Diagnosed and Underdiagnosed Illnesses ***Seaview B***
Moderator: Steven Oboler, MD
Steven A. Cumbea
Stephen C. Hunt, MD
Steven Oboler, MD

5. Occupation and Exposure History-Taking Techniques ***Seaview C***
Moderator: Susan H. Mather, MD, MPH
Melissa A. McDiarmid, MD, MPH

3:00 Break

3:30 Concurrent Sessions Continue

5:00 Adjourn

6:00– 7:00 p.m. Poster Session and Reception

Wednesday, June 4, 1997

Moderator: Susan Mather, MD

General Session ***Regency Ballroom***

8:00 am VA Mortality Study
Han K. Kang, DrPH

8:30 CDC Survey of Iowa Persian Gulf Veterans
Drue Barrett, PhD

9:00 NHRC Hospitalization Studies Among Persian Gulf Veterans
Cdr. Gregory C. Gray, MD, MPH

9:30 NHRC Study of Birth Defects Among Children of Persian Gulf Veterans
Cdr. Gregory C. Gray, MD, MPH

10:00 Break

10:30 Health Effects of Pyridostigmine Bromide Summary of Findings to Date
Col. Michael A. Dunn, MD

11:15 VA's Depleted Uranium Program
Melissa A. McDiarmid, MD, MPH

11:45 Panel Discussion
Moderator: Frances M. Murphy, MD, MPH
Drue Barrett, PhD
Col. Michael A. Dunn, MD
Cdr. Gregory C. Gray, MD
Han K. Kang, DrPH
Melissa A. McDiarmid, MD, MPH

12:30 pm Lunch

1:30 *Concurrent Sessions*

1. Occupational and Exposure History-Taking Techniques **Seaview C**

2. Answers to Commonly Asked Questions of Persian Gulf Veterans—Case Presentations and Interactive Forum **Regency Ballroom**
Moderator: Frances M. Murphy, MD, MPH
Arnold B. Gorin, MD
Frances M. Murphy, MD, MPH

3. It Takes a Village: Community Based Supportive Services for Persian Gulf Veterans and Family Members **Beacon B**
Moderator: Donald J. Rosenblum
Harry P. Becnel, PhD
Peter J. Ehlich
Robert S. Key
Norma King-Joiner
Steven Longoria
T. Patrick McGregor

4. Compensation and Pension Exams for Persian Gulf Veterans' Diagnosed and Underdiagnosed Illnesses **Beacon A**
Moderator: Steven Oboler, MD
Steven A. Cumbea
Stephen C. Hunt, MD
Steven Oboler, MD

5. DoD Incident Investigation—A Status Report **Shoreline A/B**
Moderator: John Kraemer
Lt. Col. Dee Dodson Morris

3:00 Break

3:30 Panel Discussion
Moderator: Frances M. Murphy, MD, MPH
Steven A. Cumbea
Arnold B. Gorin, MD
Susan H. Mather, MD, MPH
Robert M. White, JD

4:45	Concluding Remarks and Meeting Summary *Frances M. Murphy, MD, MPH*
5:00 pm	Evaluation/Awarding of Certificates/ Conclusion

Appendix M

Site Visit Questions

These questions should be asked of three groups of providers: primary care physicians (or nurse practitioner?) who are *not* designated Persian Gulf providers, Persian Gulf physicians/team, and specialists (need to determine if there are specialists assigned to Persian Gulf just as there are primary care physicians).

Introductory statement should be made to the effect that this is not intended to be a comprehensive survey. Rather, we are looking for ideas from front-line providers about how they view the system, how well it seems to function vis a vis the guidelines, and what they think could be done to improve the program.

Providers

1. How are patients triaged, from your point of view?

2. What type of orientation did you receive regarding this program?

3. What is your understanding of Phase I versus Phase II, that is, how do patients get referred to Phase II?

4. How do you address specific problems?
    - chronic fatigue
    - headache

- diarrhea

(for specialists, ask their area)

5. How do you define an undiagnosed condition? Would any diagnosis eliminate that patient from the category undiagnosed condition?

6. Who actually sees the patient (conducts the exam)?

7. What kind of feedback do you give the patient?
   - diagnosis
   - PG War related
   - additional options

8. How do you refer a patient to a specialist in Phase I (the PG Registry exam)? How long does it take? Are there any barriers to this?

How do you refer a patient for a Phase II exam? How long does that take? Are there any barriers to such a referral?

9. Who manages the patient medically once diagnosis is made?

10. What kind of follow-up do you receive after referral? after diagnosis? That is, do you receive feedback on what happened to the patient?

11. If the illness is deemed non-service related, is there any contact between you and the community physician caring for the patient?

12. Are there any differences between men and women in the diagnostic or referral process?

13. What do you think of the program?

14. What would you do to improve the program?

Outreach

1. Is there a designated staff member or program charged with outreach to Persian Gulf veterans regarding services available to them? Who?

2. What is the message of the outreach? (description of program, number to call, who should apply, etc.)

3. What is the facility doing with regard to community outreach for Persian Gulf veterans?
    - specific activities
    - scope of activities
    - any evaluation of the effectiveness of outreach

Intake

1. Is there a centralized intake point and/or procedure?

2. How are Persian Gulf veterans identified?

3. Once identified, how are Persian Gulf veterans informed about the program?
    - Is there a designated person at the facility to do this?
    - What is the veteran told about the program?

4. How are non-medical personnel being informed/trained regarding the Registry (written materials, workshops, etc)?

5. Who is being trained? (i.e., how is "non-medical personnel" defined?)

Access

1. How are appointments scheduled for Phase I?

2. Are there different procedures for those with and without symptoms?

3. What is the veteran told about the actual process of the exam, consultations, etc.?

Appendix N

Summary of Responses to Requests for Information

VA FACILITY RESPONSES TO UCAP

Protocol

Adequate—32: Additional Comments

• At the time the protocol was established, it did serve the purpose. After several years, however, the protocol becomes less efficient and comprehensive. Particularly after completion of Phase I, there is rarely enough to assess and complete the veteran's evaluation. More and more frequently I use Phase I and II simultaneously to achieve the diagnostic work-up. These two phases should be combined into one step.

• For female veterans, a laboratory hormonal profile and gynecology clinic evaluation should be part of the initial work-up, not part of Phase II.

• The Protocol is adequate but may be too inclusive. The initial exam documentation on "appropriate" forms is time-consuming and numerous. Phase II protocols require tests and procedures that would not all ordinarily be done on every individual. The "minimum work-ups" listed for the specific symptoms may be too invasive and in the global "risk-benefit ratio," have the potential to be too risky for the veteran.

• Recommending lumbar punctures for everyone with complaints of headaches or memory loss seems a bit extreme.

• More emphasis should be placed on the formal psychosocial assessment of veterans, especially in light of stress and its impact on an individual's medical well-being.

• Has lengthy paper work.

• Need for a psychiatric exam or clinical psychology exam to be part of the medical exam. There is also a need for a social work survey as part of the exam. We need standardized questions from headquarters.

• Consider incorporating one or more psychological screens in the protocol exam.

• Include some type of psychological screening.

• Need some means of quantifying the symptomatology because frequently patients have multiple complaints and all complaints are not equal either in severity or frequency of occurrence.

• The protocol system should facilitate the exchange of information among participating centers and physicians in a VISN in order to optimize clinical and support decision making.

• Lacks a detailed psychosocial assessment needed to thoroughly evaluate this patient group.

• For patients who have symptoms of chronic fatigue and/or sleep disorders, a sleep study would be an additional evaluation that may be indicated.

• Completion of the Phase II protocol is very time-intensive and the diagnoses, or lack thereof, seem to be of questionable value.

• The clinical protocol addresses complaints and diagnostics but not detailed history. Perhaps allowing the physician to attach pertinent history wherever applicable would help to assess the patient's concerns even though there is no diagnosis.

• The protocol does provide a general overview and resource to the examiner.

• Comprehensive and helpful. Should continue to be used without major changes. The weakness is its limitations for the diagnosis of the nature and cause(s) of the illnesses or symptoms presented. The routine examination and tests offered by this protocol are regularly found to be negative and the evaluations by specialists are diagnostically inconclusive most of the time. The diagnosis of chemically induced disease(s) involves different tests and approaches not available for routine medical practice. They should not be added to the current protocol because more disadvantages than benefits would result. But we need to speed up the research work on Gulf War veterans' illnesses.

• It would be helpful to develop algorithms to guide clinicians in ordering tests/consults to assess symptoms/conditions that are identified in the evaluation.

• For a small minority of patients complaining of damage to the immune system, a protocol for a more detailed assessment of their immune systems would be time-saving.

• Protocol would be excessive if one were to follow it verbatim rather than individualize it.

• Endoscopies and biopsies of the gastrointestinal tract and biopsies of the skin lesions of the veterans with disorders of these organ systems are underused.

• It is necessary to develop a protocol for required neuropsychiatric testing to evaluate the rate of change and frequent claims of decreased mental function.

• It would be useful to add psychological testing to the routine protocol. The routine chest X-ray is worthless and should be deleted.

• The protocol lacks specificity in several areas.

• Adherence to the protocol is time-consuming for the physician as well as the patient who must make return visits to various clinics.

• Many veterans are reluctant to discuss classified information on the questionnaire. Need an executive order declassifying all information related to toxic, biological, and/or chemical warfare agent exposure.

Implementation

Implemented and administered well—28: Additional Comments

• A common difficulty is the long waiting period for consultations or procedures. Maybe there should be an established, required time frame for all requested consults, special tests, and/or procedures, taking into account the difference in facilities.

• Have experienced some problems with timely consults from specialists. Despite the fact that the consultants have been given the required protocol, they generally use their own expertise and perform tests and procedures they think are required given the symptoms.

• A main concern relates to assessment by specialty clinics, such as neurology, which is common because of the vast number of headaches and memory loss complaints. Veterans must be referred to a distant facility (300 miles) to receive these evaluations. If the veteran is well enough to work, his or her employment interferes with keeping the appointment. There needs to be better access. For young patients with complicated problems requiring rheumatology, gastroenterology, or neurology follow-up, they just cannot keep follow-up appointments so far away. Possible solutions to these problems include offering local fee-based specialty clinic, or bringing specialists from the larger medical facilities for periodic clinics one day a month or one day every other month.

• A strength is that the Registry allows for self referral—any veteran, ill or not, can obtain examination and treatment.

• Need a fast track approach. At the first encounter the new PGW (Persian Gulf War) vet should receive information about the Registry exam and enrollment in VA's primary care clinic for potential treatment and follow-up, as well as a substantiation of claim for C&P exam purposes with the name of the veteran service officer to assist the vet. Follow-up should be through letters and newsletters.

• PGW veterans should not be treated as intrinsically different from all our other veterans who may have special needs in the VA system.

• Each VA center should identify and employ experienced, competent contact persons and physicians to serve as Environmental PGW Special Program Physicians and Advisors.

• The Registry exam should be performed ASAP before or after separation or deactivation of the individual from active duty. Should be performed by experienced personnel at a local level.

• Believe a strength of our facility is that we have established one clinic that is solely responsible for the evaluation of PG veterans who wish to be enrolled on the Registry.

• A large number of VA medical centers do not have a sleep lab to conduct sleep studies (polysomnography). Obtaining this test from the private sector is expensive, time-consuming, and delays the evaluation process. For most small- to medium-sized VAs, however, it is not cost-effective to have a sleep lab in-house. No easy solution has been identified.

• Experience a number of no-shows because a majority of vets seeking evaluations maintain full-time jobs and may live some distance from the medical center.

• Foster the idea that the PG exam is not merely one evaluation, rather it is a series of evaluations until the various diagnoses are established or discounted and other conclusions can be drawn. This may require a managed care approach where designated providers would conduct both the initial and follow-up evaluations and draw on subspecialty support when indicated.

• Promulgate and support the option of hospitalization in complex or geographically remote cases.

• There are great problems with the time and availability of specialized personnel required to conduct multiple tests and procedures before a condition can legitimately be considered "undiagnosed." Only rarely can this be accomplished with a single visit. For centers that serve an extensive geographic area, this raises the question of hospitalization.

• Have developed a worksheet to keep track of where patients are in the process and the results of their evaluations.

• Phase II has not been well implemented due to a lack of clear guidelines regarding its objectives and use. Practically speaking, to involve a large group of diverse specialists in an individual patient's care is disjointed and unproductive as the Primary Care Model is being implemented in health care.

• Because of an increase in the number of vets seeking exams and the time it takes to adequately accomplish these exams, need a full-time physician to perform PG and other environmental contaminant examinations.

• From the clinical perspective, our physicians conducting the PG exams feel that there are frequently changing directives for conducting these exams.

• Delays have been experienced in the timeliness with which consultations are obtained.

• We have had difficulties getting the affiliated medical school to complete examinations in a timely and appropriate manner. Of particular difficulty is their problem with the concept of "undiagnosed illness."

• More feedback to the examining physician after the exams are completed would be beneficial. It would allow the physician to be appraised as to any improvements he or she could make such as the acceptability of diagnosis.

• Have fully implemented the protocol.

• Because of evaluations in numerous specialty clinics, a great deal of effort must be expended to coordinate the medical information. It would be good to have the generalist staff facilitate the overview of all the specialist exams.

• Gulf War veteran satisfaction at our facility is high because the VRP is in charge of both the Registry and the return and follow-up clinics. The VRP dedicates unlimited time for these veterans. Because he or she is responsible for both the exams and the follow-up care, there is continuity of care and availability of medical assistance when needed.

• Current system is only limited by waiting times due to a lack of examiners and primary care providers.

• I believe the implementation is successful because there is a specific interdisciplinary clinic established to specifically capture this population of veterans. Concentrating PG veterans in one clinic with a specific group of providers establishes a "uniform approach to their unique concerns."

• Since not all services are available at our facility (e.g., neurology, orthopedics, MRI), the waiting period for an appointment at another VA facility is several months.

• There are limitations because of the availability of medical specialists and the need to refer to another VA facility.

Referral Centers

• There are long delays in acceptance of patients to referral centers. Several of our patients had to wait 9 months. Also, physician's assistants are the primary care givers in at least one referral center, and the veterans interpret this as a lessening in priority of the program.

• Referral centers should take a leadership role in integrating and communicating information among their local and VISN areas to standardize, process, and optimize service and research efforts.

• There is a problem accessing regional centers to discuss possible patient referrals. Calls to the telephone numbers provided frequently are not answered and there is no provision for leaving messages.

• It is very difficult to get through to the tertiary care centers for referral. They rarely get back to us, and it is very difficult to obtain copies of their examination results. This is a major annoyance to myself and my patients.

• There is a delay in the communication between the referral center and the clinic making the referral. This is due to both delay in the completion and mailing of reports from the referral center and to completed reports being received but placed in a record unbeknownst to the primary care physician.

• The consultation process with our research facility in Houston does not provide easy consultation with physicians knowledgeable in the latest aspects and research regarding Gulf War illnesses.

• Need some form of communication from the physicians and staff of the Stage 2 hospitals about their findings and diagnoses.

• It would help the Registry physicians to have the name of the contact person of the referral centers so that certain difficult cases could be referred in a timely manner.

• Referrals are tedious and difficult to accomplish with facilities far away. Consultant information is not always easily accessible for follow-up after referral. Better access to consultations and special tests should be provided and reports kept in a file separate from the general medical record. Would recommend a fast track to these centers for appropriately selected veterans.

• While the Phase I protocol is adequate for the vast majority of patients seen, about 5% require further evaluation by specialists at another facility. This presents several problems. First, inconvenience to the veteran, who is required to devote 2 to 4 days for travel and exams/tests. Another is the poor communication between the referral centers and the referring facilities. There is often no written response from the specialists or, if there is one, its receipt is greatly delayed.

• Patients who go to the referral centers must remain for a great deal of time. This concern was expressed primarily by those veterans who are employed and have families.

Other Recommendations

• Following the veteran's PG exam, an appointment should be made with his other primary care physician and a list of recommendations should be given to that physician for a workup of the veteran's complaints. If the workup does not uncover the cause of his or her complaint, the veteran should be referred to the PG physician for further evaluation and/or referral to one of the four referral centers.

• There needs to be better coordination between the Registry exam and the C&P exam to avoid duplication. Should any additional findings be uncovered during the C&P exam, they should be forwarded to the veteran's primary care physician.

• One physician in each facility should be responsible for the PG Registry for consistent, good quality evaluations.

• Need a methodology for screening-out veterans who are simply voicing symptoms that they have read about.

• No changes needed.

• Need quarterly or semi-annual review/recommendations on diagnosis and follow-up.

• Tests should be specified up front.

• Residents who are performing the PG evaluations need to be closely supervised by their attending physicians and need to be educated about possible exposures and outcomes.

• Recommendations for lab tests and X-rays should have studies completed at referral centers rather than at the parent facility so consultants might benefit from results and provide timely conclusions and recommendation.

• The physician and clerk assigned to the Persian Gulf program should be kept as a team to better address issues. At the completion of all tests and consults, the physician should review the chart for any possible omissions.

Education

• Need "in-service" training for primary health care providers and specialty clinics within the VAMC.

• An inclusive discussion, made available to VRPs, of the "alternative" explanations and proposed treatments and VA's response to those proposals would be helpful.

• There should be educational programs geared to the veterans and broadcast on local television to bring them up to date on PG health care issues.

• Education of the primary care providers in the treatment of such conditions as chronic pain, headaches, fibromyalgia, chronic fatigue syndrome, irritable bowel syndrome, and rashes would be of great benefit.

• Continuing Medical Education programs should be developed for periodic updates, as well as interfaces with new VA providers in a cooperative educational manner.

• The most important factor in the care of these patients is the role of education of the vets as to what is known about the exposures at this point in time, and reassurance that research has not shown evidence of a communicable disease or an increase in the birth defect rate. An open, informative, and compassionate attitude in dealing with these patients helps to allay fears and makes for better rapport with the patients and overall better outcome.

- Education provided to the environmental physicians through the annual national conferences, video conferences, teleconferences, and the distribution of new research and development materials has been very beneficial. However, access to this kind of information for the veteran appears to be very limited. It would be beneficial to develop an educational system utilizing newsletters, brochures, etc. to continually educate the vets regarding new developments and research studies.
- Many channels exist for the PG Registry physician to be educated about new developments, but not for the specialists who see PG vets on consult. They need education too.
- Outreach efforts should be enhanced through the VISN level by coordination among the veteran service officer, and National Guard, Reserve and active veterans' service organizations, as well as community service and employers.
- We have a very high no-show rate among PG vets and assume one of the reasons is because the vets are unable to get time off from work to come in for the exam which takes two half-day sessions. Employers must be better educated.
- Need information on the epidemiology of leishmaniasis, and the interaction, both hypothetically and practically, of cholinesterase inhibitors and insecticides and their potential for lasting neurological complications. Need a list and description of ongoing research relevant to the medical issues of PG illness(es) and abstracts on published articles.
- While the recent national meeting was excellent, the veterans and the general public have not been properly informed or prepared. The only information most of them have access to is via the news media, which is spotty, inadequate, and often distorted.
- Need to continue annual 2-day conferences. Also need to train clerical staff on the importance of clear documentation and what information is needed to assist staff in headquarters. One unified and indexed handbook to assist the clerical staff processing PG exams would be beneficial.
- Training should be continued on the clinical treatment and ongoing research studies of Persian Gulf veterans. On a local level, ongoing outreach is needed to educate agencies and vets on the registry program and other VA services.
- Veterans need to understand the purpose of the protocol exam and the Registry and the fact that it has nothing to do with claims of disability or compensation determination.

• Need short video or short closed-circuit presentation that goes over the Registry form to make sure we are complying with everything that needs to be done. It would be helpful to have information on such things as depleted uranium, microplasma, etc. to be able to respond to veterans who bring up these topics.

• Education for both providers and veterans could be improved. It would be helpful to have pamphlets available for veteran and service officer education on the purpose of the Registry. Publications and articles of interest to both veterans and providers need to be available in the treatment areas.

• Providers of primary care need to be better informed as to new information that would assist them in treating PG vets. An annual presentation coordinated by the PG physician at each station would be a valuable contribution.

• Continue education via yearly national conference, live satellite conferences, and regular relay of current publications/articles.

• The physician and clerk assigned to the Persian Gulf program should be properly trained.

• Veterans need to be better informed about the workup and referral process, that is, only unexplained cases are referred to Houston facility.

• Need a "fact sheet" published quarterly that separates facts from media reporting.

• One way to alleviate concern may be to frequently communicate with all veterans via newsletter so that they will not be confused by the conflicting reports in the press.

• The VA could have seminars that would keep physicians who do the Registry exams abreast of new developments.

• After 5 years of the program, it may be time to compile a current manual for the program with information such as the purpose of and eligibility for the program, exam protocols with lab and X-ray requirements, coding sheets, and sample follow-up letters.

• Outreach programs or new letters should provide the results of studies that are reassuring, such as the information regarding birth defects.

• VA personnel turnover creates difficulties for maintaining a well-informed staff that understands PG issues and eligibility.

• Efforts to provide education and outreach are fine.

• Persian Gulf program in Long Beach was excellent.

• Need medical education on medical and industrial toxicology given the concerns and question of PG veterans relating to exposures to various chemical agents.

• Providers and support staff need up-to-date information on the latest developments in Persian Gulf illnesses. The continuing medical education credit is good and needs to continue.

• Perhaps a brief training film or program similar to the one produced for the ex-POW protocol program would be useful for orienting new staff.

• Teleconferences and educational conferences have been extremely beneficial in keeping providers aware of the current status of research and in helping to defuse the multiple myths surrounding this complex problem.

• Insufficient work has been done in educating providers other than the PG providers about the clinical protocol and Gulf War health issues. The annual conference on Gulf War health consequences is excellent. Unfortunately, access is limited. The organization and planning of conferences and workshops to be held within each VISN would offer greater opportunities for other providers.

• Overall implementation has been quite successful due to the continuing education efforts by VA headquarters.

• While Persian Gulf providers have been educated well, other staff—and particularly residents—who are affiliated with VA medical centers have not had the benefit of that education. They and the staff who are not directly involved in the program but who regularly see Persian Gulf patients need to be more familiar with the program, the current research and understanding on the illnesses of PG vets, and how best to met the needs of these veterans.

• Education for PG-designated providers is great, but there needs to be more education at the local level so that other clinicians who treat PG veterans in their practices may learn about recent research and medical management updates.

• Each facility needs to improve the awareness of the providers, other staff, and veterans on PG issues.

• It would be good to have a succinct one-page monthly update to hand out to providers who do exams and care.

• Providers have indicated they would like the Persian Gulf Review and news releases from the central VA to be sent directly to them so as to reduce any delay in receiving this information.

• There is a tremendous need to educate all the physicians involved with the veterans' care concerning Persian Gulf medical issues. Often we use our consultants for the completion of the exams. By educating the providers, they would become more sensitive toward those Persian Gulf issues and subsequently could address the requirements of the examination and the patient's needs.

• Need more publicity about the nature and current findings of ongoing epidemiologic studies for veterans.

• Some veterans are unaware that they could return for further care.

Problems

• Primary care physicians are, for the most part, unaware of the Persian Gulf Registry.

• The issue of compensation clouds the efforts to collect objective information for the Registry. Need a greater collaborative effort between VAHS R&D and the VBA to ensure this distinction is understood by the veteran.

• Several veterans have become disillusioned with the care they have been offered and have given up on the system. Some have had worsening problems but have failed to return for reevaluation.

• The VA program lacks focus. When there is no well-defined disease entity or broadly defined clinical syndrome(s), and no etiologic specificity, identified with any degree of certainty, there is an unhappy doctor- (provider-) patient relationship.

• Frustrated at not being able to address all concerns voiced by the PG vets because there are no definitive answers.

• Considered not necessarily as a weakness but rather as a continuing challenge/opportunity for improvements is how best the provider can convey to the veterans' satisfaction the findings/explanations of their illnesses or the health consequences of Gulf War service in light of continuing media interest and reports that at times contain conflicting information.

• Our follow-up letters, which are required by central VA, prominently state that the purpose is to give veterans a brief clinical summary of exam findings. However, a number of veterans interpreted the letters to be a denial of compensation benefits. We were told to stop sending out the letters.

• "Undiagnosed illness" is very difficult. Providers are very uncomfortable with the formal diagnosis of "undiagnosed illness." Something like "Insufficient clinical evidence at present to warrant a diagnosis of any acute or chronic pathologic condition or residuals thereof" would be better.

• Not so subtle pressure to make a diagnosis of a chronic pathologic condition has resulted in somewhat a "Catch 22" situation for the examiners. If a diagnosis of a chronic pathologic conditions can be made at the time of re-evaluation and the symptoms relating to that condition were not present while the veteran was on active duty or within 12 months of discharge, then the veteran may well have service-connection reduce or severed.

• Providing updated, ongoing information to dozens of staff physicians as well as a large group of residents in training has proven to be both difficult and spotty.

• Too many Persian Gulf war veterans do not understand there is a registry for all who served.

• The percentage of no-shows is high.

• We saw a veteran with alleged exposure to depleted uranium and sent urine samples to the depleted-uranium program in Baltimore but have had difficulty receiving the results of the urine tests. Maybe they could be made available through email to the respective physicians.

• A major weakness of program involves difficulty in diagnosis, that is the Persian Gulf syndrome is not a well-defined process. Veterans and the mass media continue to allege that "something is being hidden" from the public by authorities, which makes dealing with veterans somewhat difficult.

• Have not discerned exposures that have been reasonably linked with the myriad health concerns presented by patients.

• This entire process is becoming politicized like the Agent Orange program.

• This program, as presented to the veterans—as a potential source of monetary compensation—has created unrealistic expectations and has probably biased some of the veterans presenting histories that is thereby making the use of such information for statistical data collection questionable.

• The true workload associated with these examinations and corresponding data recording requirements is not being captured or allowed for.

• The waiting period for a Persian Gulf Registry evaluation, return, and follow-up clinic is several months, but the physician in charge resolves this by overbooking.

• There are ongoing problems with identification of in-theater PG veterans. It is difficult to determine eligibility accurately using the DHCP system. There need to be two designations—"Persian Gulf Service" and "Persian Gulf era."

• Funds for biopsy of lesions and testing for toxins, neuropsychological testing, or genetic testing have not been made available at the local level. Generally speaking, it is hoped that the clinical program will be expanded. As more information comes to light about toxic exposure to combustion materials from crude oil fumes, biological and/or chemical warfare agents and exposures to and effects of vaccines and depleted uranium, the testing program for veterans must also be expanded.

Persian Gulf Registry Code Sheet/Data

• For sleep studies, a column should be designated to reflect the results from such an evaluation.

• Forms required for use in documentation of PG exams are ambiguous. The ICD-9 codes required for the documentation form are not specific for symptoms, but rather diagnoses. Yet they are required for each symptom. At the end of the exam, the veteran must assist in delineating which ICD-9 code for which symptom is to be listed as the most severe, and only one must be selected. Often this is difficult, as several symptoms cause the veteran concern. At the end of the form the provider must decide if the veteran has an unexplained problem or illness, but there are no formal guidelines to follow. It might be better to ask whether all the veteran's symptoms can be treated with current therapies.

• There is no computerized data collection sheet. The present PG form is mainly for statistical purposes. A proper form for a history and physical exam should be added.

• Since many of the specialty exams are performed as part of Phase I in order to arrive at a final diagnosis that is coded in the Phase I section, the completion of the Phase II part of the protocol is then very problematic. We have recently tried to review these exams at 3 and 6 months to see if a Phase II coding sheet can reasonably be completed and then resubmitted. We have uniformly found that the clinic physicians do not understand the requirements of completing the code sheets.

• Persian Gulf Registry code sheet question 26 for diagnostic consultations is difficult to answer. This question requests information about consultation referral and diagnosis. The diagnosis is made by the consultant and therefore is not known at the time of the Phase I registry exam. The feedback the examiners have received from the veterans is that few of the questions on the form are difficult to understand. Veterans frequently have questions about the definition of the terms "petrochemical" and "microwaves" (questions 18J, 18P).

• The code sheet (Section 25 A/J, Column 3) mentions specifically the month and year of onset of symptoms. An "if available" in parentheses should be present after the month to simplify the process.

• Some veterans have difficulty converting responses on their part of the code sheet to numerical values. They need guidance.

• The separation of the examination protocol into phases is clumsy, inefficient (redundant), and unnecessarily confusing. Specifically, this relates to the reiteration of diagnoses, ad nauseum, in the two phases. Phase II, item 26 numerical categories have always been confusing, both in this protocol and that for the Agent Orange. They are subject to different interpretations and lead to confused data.

• The information in the Registry exam or the military CCEP must be a part of the consolidated medical record and should be made available with the service record to the evaluating C&P or treating site physician. The Austin Data Center should provide the treatment center with periodic feedback regarding the exam.

• The VA should capture the vets' special program needs through a national database at the time a VA card for service is issued. This data screen should reflect the veterans, status, PGW, RVN, POW, VIS, C&P pending, SC, female veteran, or other (i.e., radiation, Bosnia, etc.).

Items of Note

- Compensation and pension physicians are providing Phase I exams at the same time as C&P exams in one VA.
- Frances Murphy and her staff have been most helpful.
- One suggestion from a VA is as follows: "...it may be more cost effective to eliminate the Persian Gulf exam program and treat their medical problems like [those of] any other patient. The one aspect of the exam program that provided significant assistance to the Persian Gulf veterans and their families was the Social Worker..." who is no longer funded.
- Guidance from headquarters has been outstanding.
- The approach of the VA should be to give credence to the complaints of PGW veterans.

VETERANS' SERVICE ORGANIZATIONS RESPONSES TO UCAP

Thirty-seven letters were sent to Veterans' Service Organizations (VSOs) with details on the IOM committee on the UCAP. The letter requested the VSOs to comment on the adequacy of the protocol and its implementation as well as the need for education of providers and veterans. Five responses were received, and are summarized below.

I. PROTOCOL

A. Overall Comments

- The protocol is adequate to assess and address the wide range of veterans' illnesses (1).
- The VA needs to examine the possibility of depleted uranium exposure as a cause of illness in Persian Gulf War veterans.
- Further assessment should be done on the health of the veterans' families.

B. Medical Histories

- Less emphasis should be placed on the veterans' history of smoking.
- More information should be included in the histories to elicit a detailed history of the extent of the veterans' exposures to various hazardous agents.

C. Exams

- Cease the use of urinalysis for depleted-uranium testing and tell all previously tested vets that their results were probably inaccurate.
- Doctors should conduct standard clinical testing for fatigue, the most common complaint of Persian Gulf War veterans.
- Many of the protocol tests are improperly performed and interpreted.

D. Diagnosis

- The protocol is designed only to find common and easily detected problems. It is not adequate for detecting, assessing, or treating exposure to low-level chemical agents, biological agents, depleted uranium, etc.
- The protocol often has inconclusive results, and veterans are treated for each symptom, rather than for an illness.
- Less emphasis should be placed on stress and posttraumatic stress disorder (PTSD) as diagnoses.

E. Treatment

- Should PTSD patients be treated differently from other mentally ill patients?
- There is little evidence that the VA is effectively treating veterans.

F. Implementation

- Many facilities were slow to be educated on the UCAP and slower to implement the protocol.
- Veterans in the protocol should be assigned to a primary care physician to oversee all phases of testing and treatment.
- Information on subsequent specialty consults does not get back to the physician who conducted the original Registry exam.

  - National referral centers (NRCs) should be able to diagnose patients, but often do not fulfill that duty. Furthermore, only 1,000 veterans have been referred, and over 13,000 do not have a diagnosis.
  - NRCs need to have specific teams assigned to provide Phase II exams.
  - VISNs should be made able to handle Phase II exams because veterans often have difficulty getting to an NRC.

II. EDUCATION AND OUTREACH

A. Veterans

- Not enough spouses and dependents are aware of, or have taken advantage of, Registry exams.
- VHA does not inform vets about new efforts in the Registry.
- Many veterans would not have known about the Registry without the veterans' service organizations.
- Veterans should be educated by VA about what exposures in the Gulf could be hazardous.

B. VA Personnel

- The VA needs a better understanding of possible toxic exposures.
- The VA needs to stop relying on information from the Department of Defense, which has proven to be inaccurate before.
- Some believe Registry providers seem to be concerned and dedicated. Others see a lack of information and interest on the part of the physicians.
- VA should consider new tests identified by non-VA groups that could help the veteran.
- Many VA physicians do not have access to the most recent medical information—the veterans often have to educate their physicians on recent developments.

    - Physicians need to put current medical knowledge into practice.
    - Many of the health care providers are first-year residents or physicians' assistants. The VA should have more experienced doctors. Inexperienced doctors are less likely to recognize difficult-to-diagnose illnesses.
    - VA staff often generate more health hazards to the veterans by continuing harmful actions such as imposing fumes from chlorine and other agents on the veterans in the facilities.

III. ADDITIONAL COMMENTS

- An independent organization should investigate the cause of veterans' illnesses.
- The VA should conduct formal outcome studies on the effectiveness of medical treatments.

- The VA should evaluate the merits of the current UCAP Phase I and Phase II systems and consider allowing VISNs to complete Phase II exams.
- Veterans often complain about insensitive physicians, ineffective care, bad follow-up, and a feeling that they are slipping through the cracks.
- The quality of care at different centers varies widely.

Appendix O

Questions Related to Traumatic Exposure

1. How many times did you see someone dying or being killed?

2. How many times did you see dead bodies of enemy soldiers?

3. How many times did you see bizarre disfigurement of bodies that resulted from wounds?

4. Did you lose a close friend in the war?

5. Did you observe anything you would consider excessively violent or brutal, even for wartime, such as mistreatment of prisoners or mutilation of bodies?

6. Did you participate in anything you would consider excessively violent or brutal, even for wartime?

7. Were you ever physically forced to have sex while deployed?

8. Were you ever sexually molested (touched or fondled) against your will while deployed?

9. Did you ever feel that you were being harassed sexually while deployed?

Please describe any other experiences that occurred during deployment in the Persian Gulf that you found extremely stressful and/or upsetting.

What was the single most upsetting thing that happened to you while you were deployed in the Gulf?

Appendix P

Patient Satisfaction

You were recently evaluated as part of the Veterans' Administration (VA) special program for diagnosis of Persian Gulf veterans' health problems. We are interested in finding out about your experiences with the care you received as part of this special program. Please take a few moments to answer the following questions regarding your impressions of, and satisfaction with, the services you received.

Getting an Appointment

1. How did you first find out about the special Persian Gulf program at the VA?

    [ ] Newspaper
    [ ] Letter sent to me
    [ ] From my local VA facility
    [ ] Friends or fellow veterans
    [ ] Other, please explain______________________________________
    ____

2. Were you able to schedule your first clinic appointment as soon as you wanted?

    [ ] Yes
    [ ] No

3. From the time you first contacted the VA and informed them that you wished to participate in the special Persian Gulf program, how long did it take before you were first seen?

[ ] Less than 2 weeks
[ ] 2 weeks to less than 1 month
[ ] 1 to 3 months
[ ] More than 3 months

4. Was the VA facility where you had your first Persian Gulf examination convenient for you to get to?

[ ] Yes
[ ] No

Clinic Visits

5. How many appointments were scheduled for you? ____________________

6. Were you able to keep all appointments scheduled for you?

[ ] Yes
[ ] No. If no, please briefly explain why____________________________

____

7. How long did it take to complete the entire evaluation for your health problems?

[ ] Less than 2 weeks (if your evaluation was completed during the first visit, check this box)
[ ] 2 weeks to less than 1 month
[ ] 1 to 3 months
[ ] More than 3 months. Please enter number of months here _________
[ ] My evaluation has not been completed.

8. Did any of your visits take place at more than one VA facility?

[ ] Yes
[ ] No

9. Are you continuing to receive health care services from the VA?

[ ] Yes, I am continuing with the special Persian Gulf program.
[ ] Yes, I have completed the special Persian Gulf program, but am continuing to receive services which were recommended to me during the Persian Gulf examinations.
[ ] Yes, I am continuing to receive services from the VA but they are not related to the special Persian Gulf program.
[ ] No

In the Provider's Office

10. Did you understand the purpose of the special VA program for Persian Gulf veterans when you arrived for your first appointment?

[ ] Yes
[ ] No

If No, to question 10, did the people at the VA facility explain the purpose of the program to you when you arrived for your appointment?

[ ] Yes
[ ] No

11. Did the provider evaluating you listen to what you had to say?

[ ] Yes, completely
[ ] Yes, somewhat
[ ] No
[ ] I had nothing to discuss

12. Did this provider take you seriously?

[ ] Yes, completely
[ ] Yes, somewhat
[ ] No

13. Did this provider seem knowledgeable about Gulf War-related symptoms?

[ ] Yes, completely
[ ] Yes, somewhat
[ ] No

14. Did you have confidence and trust in the provider you saw?

[ ] Yes, completely
[ ] Yes, somewhat
[ ] No. Please explain why not____

____

15. Did the provider explain why you needed tests in a way you could understand?

[ ] Yes, completely
[ ] Yes, somewhat
[ ] No
[ ] I did not need any tests

16. After tests were done, did the provider explain the results in a way you could understand?

[ ] Yes, completely
[ ] Yes, somewhat
[ ] Somewhat
[ ] Not at all
[ ] Did not need an explanation
[ ] Did not yet get results
[ ] Did not need any tests

17. Did the provider evaluating you recommend any test or other procedures which you did not receive?

[ ] Yes
[ ] No

If Yes to question 17, what was the reason you did not receive the recommended test(s)?

[ ] I am still waiting to have the test(s) completed
[ ] I chose not to have the test(s) done even though they were recommended
[ ] It is not convenient for me to have the test(s)
[ ] Other. Please explain ______________________________

____

18. Did the provider you saw seem to think that your symptoms were due to: (Check ALL that apply)

[ ] A medical problem related to service in the Gulf War
[ ] A medical problem *not* related to service in the Gulf War
[ ] A psychological problem related to service in the Gulf War
[ ] A psychological problem *not* related to service in the Gulf War
[ ] "Stress"
[ ] Provider didn't know
[ ] Other. Please explain ______________________________

____

Overall Impressions

19. Please rate your satisfaction with various aspects of the health care you received as part of the VA special Persian Gulf program.

A. At your local VA

very unsatisfied very satisfied

B. At the regional VA referral center [ ] Not applicable

very unsatisfied very satisfied

C. At the Persian Gulf VA referral center [ ] Not applicable

very unsatisfied very satisfied

D. From the providers who first evaluated you at your local VA

very unsatisfied very satisfied

E. From the specialists or consultants whom you have seen during any part of your evaluation at any facility in the special Persian Gulf program
[ ] Not applicable

very unsatisfied very satisfied

20. If you could have free care outside the VA for your health problems, would you choose to go to the VA again?

Definitely would not Definitely would

21. Have you sought an evaluation from a health care provider outside the VA for what you believe to be Persian Gulf-related health problems?

[ ] Yes
[ ] No

If yes to question 21, please indicate the type of provider (check ALL that apply)

[ ] Personal doctor

[ ] A doctor who I learned about and who was interested in problems related to the Persian Gulf

[ ] A health care provider other than a physician. Please describe______

____

22. Would you prefer to receive care for your problems outside the VA system?

[ ] Yes

[ ] No